The Health Collection

provided by

Genesis Health Services

Foundation

OREN LIEBERMANN

the insulin express

ONE BACKPACK, FIVE CONTINENTS, AND THE DIABETES DIAGNOSIS THAT
changed everything

FOREWORD BY DR. SANJAY GUPTA

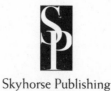

Skyhorse Publishing

Skyhorse Publishing books may be purchased in bulk at special discounts for sales promotion, corporate gifts, fund-raising, or educational purposes. Special editions can also be created to specifications. For details, contact the Special Sales Department, Skyhorse Publishing, 307 West 36th Street, 11th Floor, New York, NY 10018 or info@skyhorsepublishing.com.

Skyhorse® and Skyhorse Publishing® are registered trademarks of Skyhorse Publishing, Inc.®, a Delaware corporation.

Visit our website at www.skyhorsepublishing.com.

10 9 8 7 6 5 4 3 2 1

Library of Congress Cataloging-in-Publication Data is available on file.

Cover design by Jenny Zemanek
Cover photo credit: iStock

Print ISBN: 978-1-5107-1848-7
Ebook ISBN: 978-1-5107-1849-4

Printed in the United States of America

Contents

The names of some locations and people have been changed.

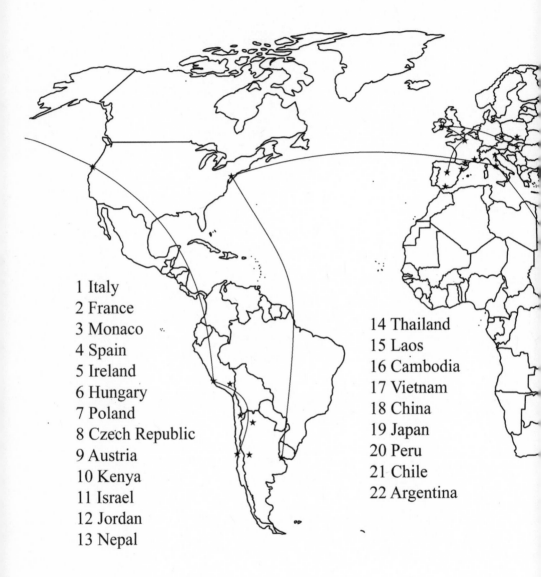

1 Italy
2 France
3 Monaco
4 Spain
5 Ireland
6 Hungary
7 Poland
8 Czech Republic
9 Austria
10 Kenya
11 Israel
12 Jordan
13 Nepal

14 Thailand
15 Laos
16 Cambodia
17 Vietnam
18 China
19 Japan
20 Peru
21 Chile
22 Argentina

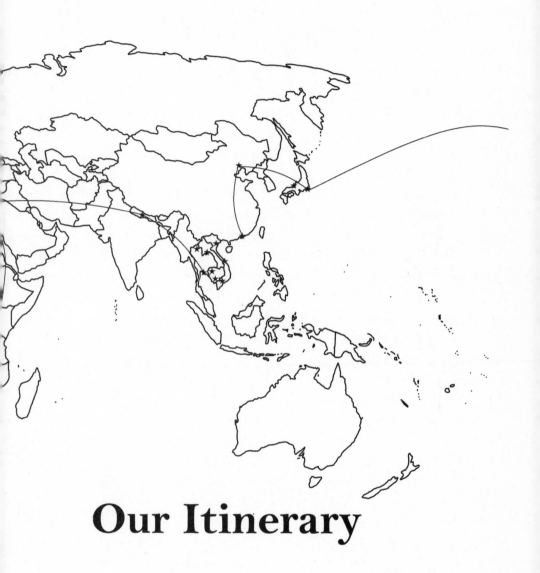

Our Itinerary

Foreword

As doctors, we often get only fleeting snapshots in time of our patients' lives. They arrive in our clinics, emergency wards, and operating rooms at the culmination of the most important physical and emotional journey of their lives. They are sick, vulnerable, and suddenly reduced to a blurry mess of lab values, imaging results, and diagnoses. It can be disorienting and humbling for the patients and their families.

Understandably, the physician's focus is on the immediate threat and how best to deal with it. Still, we rarely get a full appreciation of the incredible story and background that brought the patient to us in the first place. The fact is, we can diagnose our patient as ill, but do not fully appreciate why or how it happened. This is a missing link in the practice of medicine that my colleague Oren Liebermann brilliantly uncovers with *The Insulin Express*. He provides an incredible backstory to the germination of his own malady. It is true that we know more than ever about the physical impact of diabetes, but Oren wants us to know the emotional toll, as well.

As I started to read *The Insulin Express*, I devoured the clues about the beginning symptoms of his illness. With a journalist's diligence, no detail was too small or unimportant. It was his fastidious journaling throughout a year of triumphs and letdowns which provided the exhilarating spine to his book. As he was trekking through Nepal and climbing toward Annapurna Base Camp, I felt like I was right there with him—concerned for his welfare and wondering why he shed 45 pounds, leaving him continuously exhausted. I could peer up the final 300 steps he needed to climb, even as his body was literally breaking down and devouring itself. I silently urged him to turn back, but cheered at the photo of his success, his blood soaked with sugar.

If you have diabetes, or face any sort of challenge, *The Insulin Express* is the dose of inspiration you need to be reminded of what is possible.

It is not too often that a writer with the candor, biting sarcasm, and narrative style of Oren Lieberman writes a book so deeply personal. At first, *The Insulin Express* is a sweeping travelogue of a man who was born to travel and who sacrifices a great deal to do so. Oren writes with the irreverence and brisk pace of the world traveler he set out to be. Again, striking details are never omitted, but there is a relentless nature to his narrative, as he candidly shares his entry into the world of journalism and the resulting trials along the way. It is about relationships with friends, colleagues, and new loves.

It is also, however, an anatomy of an illness that leaves him with the option of possibly dying in a dusty, remote Nepalese clinic, or coming out the other side stronger and more inspired than before. We will all have challenges in our lives; even the most blessed among us. It is not the challenge upon which we will reflect in our later years, however, but how we behaved in the face of those obstacles. And, for that, Oren has valuable lessons to share with all his readers.

"Deep within all of us lies the truth." This is the note I scribbled halfway through the book. On some subconscious level, Oren likely knew what was happening deep within his body even if his brain, like all of ours, is wired for denial. And in there lies one of the lessons. The stories of our patients, chock full of details, provide not only a wonderful narrative, but also critical insights into ourselves—if we just take the time to share and listen.

—Dr. Sanjay Gupta, Chief Medical Correspondent for CNN

Preface

I had always wanted to write a book. I never quite knew what book it was that I would write, but that seemed less important than the actual intent to write it. The story would sort itself out once I put pen to paper. (When I was in fourth grade, I wrote the first four pages of a novel. It was one of the longest things I had ever written. I showed it to my dad, who pointed out that it had a lot of curse words. I was writing an adult novel, I reasoned, and adults curse.)

Suffice it to say this is certainly not the book I thought I would write. I had always dreamt of writing a book about my life as a test pilot. I hate to break it to my younger self, but this is not that book.

When we started traveling, I had a vague notion that I wanted to write a book about the trip. What I couldn't figure out was why my story was compelling. On Valentine's Day 2014, the day I was officially diagnosed with diabetes, I got my answer.

Since then, I have vowed to spend every Valentine's Day overseas as a way of reminding myself—and my disease—who's in charge here.

This is my life, just as certainly as your life is your own, and I will not have my decisions dictated to me by diabetes. I hope you find similar inspiration somewhere within these pages.

Chapter 1

June 13, 2011
31°47′05.8″N 35°12′57.0″E
Jerusalem

The Aussies are drunk again.

For a fourth straight night, they consume an ungodly amount of alcohol—mostly beer, but occasionally they mix in something more potent for variety, perhaps a vodka or licorice arak. They are waging war on their livers, attacking with wave upon wave of alcoholic beverage. Since we're in Jerusalem, I can only assume this is a holy war, though what deity they fight for or what set of beliefs they proselytize I have not yet divined. They drink with the fervor and fanaticism of Crusaders, except instead of trying to rid the Middle East of one particular religious group or another, they are trying to vanquish the alcohol supply here.

Based on what I remember of Mrs. Bejda's tenth grade biology class, their livers are bound to give up at some point. They must, anatomically speaking, suffer alcohol poisoning eventually. But I see no signs of such mortal weakness. They drink with a swagger and confidence that is uniquely Australian, confident that tomorrow will come no matter what conglomeration of drinks they imbibe.

Nico seems to be the ringleader. Tall and brunette, she is incredibly fun and, somehow, in very good shape. Her sinewy arms and legs remind me of an Olympic high jumper armed with a trigger-happy smile. She has trained her body to metabolize grain alcohol into pure muscle, a trick I remind myself to learn. Nico's fitness hides her age—she could be anywhere between twenty-five and forty—old enough to have built up a resistance to the deleterious effects of alcohol, yet young enough to ignore them (though I suspect she is closer to our late twenties). She is gregariously loud and laughs between frequent sips of booze. My fiancée, Cassie, and I like her instantly.

Sim—short for Simeon—is her partner in crime. Also tall and lean, but much quieter and more laid-back. He sports cropped dirty blond hair and a boyishly short beard. Nothing bothers him. I suspect he is a good surfer, no matter what his blood-alcohol content. He stays with Nico on every drink. Claire, the final member of Team Aussie on this night, is shorter, quieter, and perhaps inwardly confident that there is a limit to how much one should drink in a night and maybe we crossed that limit a few hours back, somewhere between the third beer and fourth shot.

The three Australians have been traveling for months, working their way across parts of Asia and the Middle East.

"We smashed Jordan," says Nico, laughing.

"Yeah, definitely," Sim agrees.

"Absolutely smashed Jordan."

"Smashed?" I ask, quite sure that no one has taken an oversized sledgehammer or other such destructive device to the Hashemite Kingdom in recent days. Now that I am on vacation, I have no reason to keep up with the news, but I feel like that one would've come to my attention.

"Oh, right, sorry," Nico says. "*Smashing* is getting really pissed somewhere. Really, really drunk. We smashed Jordan." She and Sim lapse into giggles, as if remembering a covert first kiss or an embarrassing secret.

"I thought Jordan didn't have any alcohol."

"It doesn't. We found a place that let us drink in a back room with no windows so no one could see us."

I don't whistle in appreciation of their commitment to finding booze, but I should. There are no limits to how far they will go to drink. Their daily routine is like clockwork. I could set my watch by the time they wake up hungover, find breakfast, hydrate, then get back to drinking. The only variable in their day that I observe is the time they pass out at night. I suspect even this can be reduced to a quantifiable formula through the calculus of alcoholic absorption into the bloodstream based on what they drink, how fast they drink it, and how long they wait in between drinks. Most nights the answers are beer, fast, and not at all.

They don't bother with the tediousness of seeing the sites of Jerusalem. Who cares about the site where Jesus was betrayed if you can check out the pub where Judas drank afterward? The Western Wall and the Dome of the Rock, a mere fifteen-minute walk from our hostel, mean far less to them than Carlsberg and Maccabi beer. The Church of the Holy Sepulchre, the City of David—these are all insignificant. You can read about them later in a tour book or see them online. With today's broadband speed and accessibility, you can have a high-resolution image of these sites or an HD video on your smartphone in seconds. Besides, the holy sites aren't going anywhere. The beer is. They have drunk their way through half the world, and now they are steadily working on the other half.

I am impressed. I have never seen such single-minded determination to do one thing and one thing alone, even when surrounded with so many other options. When Sir Edmund Hillary was climbing Everest for the first time, all he could really do was go up. When Neil Armstrong was on his way to the moon, he had no choice but to proceed. Here the Aussies have a whole country full of things they've never seen or done, and yet they focus the sum of their not inconsiderable energies on the imbibing of distilled and fermented spirits. Their BAC must be somewhere north of completely shit-faced, but here they are, cackling and chatting their way through another half-liter of sub-par Israeli beer.

The peer pressure is enormous, even if completely unintentional. They don't need me to drink with them, but I join the fun and drink anyway, knowing full well they are seasoned veterans at this, while I wallow in my newly discovered amateur status.

Once I tried to keep up with a friend of mine who could easily hold down more booze than I could. Mitch was a high school friend whom I hadn't seen since long before we both turned twenty-one. He always outweighed me by a good forty pounds, and at our friend's wedding I learned exactly how much he could outdrink me too. The groom found me twenty minutes later, lying face up on a sidewalk next to a puddle of my evacuated stomach contents. When Cassie came looking for me, he jovially informed her that he had called me a cab. Cassie was livid, first at my sorry state, and second at the fact that my state forced the groom to call me a cab. Any mention that I was being tried twice for the same crime and that constitutional amendments have, for centuries, prohibited double jeopardy would've earned me a swift and severe ass-kicking. I kept my mouth shut and accepted the verbal lacerations as fair punishment.

Maybe it wouldn't have been so bad if I hadn't screwed up so colossally the next morning. We had an early flight back home. I dropped Cassie off at check-in, then went to return our rental car. In that ten-minute difference, she made the flight and I didn't. I somehow found a way to feel worse than my hangover. To top it off, the entire groom's family was on my flight, and they knew exactly what had happened.

I push those fleeting thoughts aside as I keep up with the Aussies. One must never think of the past while halfway through an all-night drinking session.

In between rounds of whatever alcohol happens to be the cheapest at the moment, I begin to pick up some Australian. Theoretically, they speak English Down Under, but to my American ears, they speak a dialect of English that uses enough new words and phrases to qualify as its own language.

"You piked last night," Nico yells at Sim.

"I did not pike!" Sim retorts.

"Yes, you did, you piker."

"I am not a piker!"

"What the hell is piking?" I manage to interject.

I learn that piking is calling it a night early, or worse, not going out at all. Pikers are "tired" or "sleepy" or "want to stay in"—all very anti-Down Under concepts from what I can tell. Peer pressure and a steady barrage of insults are the best weapons against piking. "You better not fucking pike!" or "You piker! You piked last night too!" are all good sentences to keep on standby to ward off even the merest thought of piking.

I dare not pike.

Not even when I have a damn good reason to pike. Cassie and I signed up for a tour of Masada, Ein Gedi, and the Dead Sea that leaves at 3 a.m. so we can climb the snake path to Masada before sunrise.

For us, this vacation is a bit of a celebration—I proposed to Cassie two weeks ago on the morning of her graduation from graduate school—and we're trying to pack in as much sightseeing as possible between trips to visit my family. Cassie was more than a bit surprised to see a ring in the small box in which I had promised to put earrings, and I was more than a bit relieved to finally unweave the web of very delicate lies I had spun to cover both my repeated trips to New York City's diamond district and the gaping hole in my savings account.

This is Cassie's inaugural journey to Israel, which makes it her first time meeting my cousins, since only my immediate family emigrated to the States. One side of my family greets her with open arms, eager to meet an upcoming addition to the Liebermann clan. The other side spends three hours trying to convince me to call off the engagement simply because Cassie isn't Jewish. The conversation is distinctly one-sided, partly because I know that arguing won't change anyone's opinion, but mostly because I don't speak Hebrew well enough to explain to them the lunacy of their own position. Yet I understand it just fine.

They cite texts written more than a few millennia ago and spout scripture they insist be interpreted literally and without the slightest taint of modernity. Their attempts to dissuade me from attending my own upcoming nuptials involve phrases like "silent Holocaust," which is apparently the theoretical murder of future Jewish children by marrying outside the faith, and they compare my love for Cassie to my love for ice pops, since, according to their strict Orthodox ethos, a relationship with a *goy* can't contain real emotion. I allow the conversation to last three hours only because that's how long I can ignore their incessant psychobabble while I try to remember the days when I enjoyed their company.

After we rid ourselves of their fundamentalist monologues, we get back to exploring the country where I spent my earliest years. We booked the Masada excursion months ago, and we've been looking forward to it as one of the highlights of our trip.

Surprisingly, the Aussies have decided to venture out and explore a bit, taking a short break from the only activity in which they have shown an active and unyielding interest. They have signed up for the same tour. The drive to Masada will take about an hour, not nearly long enough to catch up on the sleep that we are so willfully sacrificing in the name of Dionysus. This fact stumbles across our subconscious, but we push it down into the darkest recesses of our id for a few more drinks.

We give in to some combination of exhaustion and intoxication late in the evening. Leaving the last shreds of our sobriety at the bar behind us, we head to bed, letting our circadian rhythms figure out what to do with the few hours of sleep we will get before a day in the desert sun.

We stumble onto the tourist bus a few hours later, all of us groggy and perhaps a bit hungover. More than a bit. The streets of Jerusalem are still dark as we make our way into the Negev desert. The bus rumbles to a stop at Masada, and we begin climbing the winding path up the side of the plateau to the ancient Roman fortress on top.

Once again, I am impressed. Our new friends are awesome. They probably have no future and can't remember the past, but they are awesome. They are the very definition of living in the present. Nico, Claire, and Sim fly up the trail as if they are well-rested and hydrated. They are neither, but that doesn't stop them. A forty-five-minute hike takes them twenty-five minutes. If I didn't know better, I would swear they borrowed jet-powered skates from Wile E. Coyote.

We watch sunrise from the top of Masada as the first rays of light hit the Dead Sea. It is an awesome place to take in the dawn. Deserts are generally not considered particularly beautiful places, but the Negev absolutely is. The barren plateaus and jagged rock formations stretch into the distance, revealing a harsh landscape that makes survival a challenge for every living creature, including the recently inebriated. The sun inches its way up the desert sky, laboriously pushing its way through the morning haze in waves of red and orange. The sky is ablaze, and its reflection off the crystal-clear waters of the Dead Sea leaves us staring at the bands of light as they grow brighter and deeper.

Moments after we see the sun, we feel its heat. The temperature skyrockets after sunrise. Beads of sweat make their way from my exposed head down my face and into my eyes, before they are collected in a sopping mess in my increasingly wet shirt. We soon make our way off the exposed mound of King Herod's ancient city to find shade and water.

Our bus takes us to Ein Gedi, an oasis in the middle of the desert, and then to the Dead Sea. All the while, the sun beats down on us. Waves of heat feel like physical weights on our backs. The desert sun in the midst of summer is at full force, the firecracker explosion of its heat directed right at us.

On our way back to Jerusalem, red spots appear on Cassie's arms, as if a colony of ravenous fire ants had scrambled over her skin and bit her all over. Cassie fights the urge to scratch. Whatever it is, scratching won't help. The spots spread to her back as the apparently invisible fire ants keep attacking. To me, it looks a bit like poison ivy, but I know that's impossible since there is no poison ivy anywhere near us—not in Israel and certainly not in the Negev desert. Our best guess is that it's the sun. Too much exposure, and Cassie's body is not handling it well. The hives cover a growing part of her back, neck, and arms.

Two things are immediately apparent. We need some kind of medication. And we're going to have to pike.

We rummage through our makeshift first aid kit, imagining what Cassie would look like if we covered all of the spots with bandages. No amount of opening, searching, and closing our little kit will change the fact that we don't have serious allergy medication.

We venture across the hall to the hostel dorm room the Aussies share.

"Hey guys, we can't go out tonight," I say to Nico as she merrily opens the door. "Cassie broke out in hives, and they're not going away."

Nico studies the spots for a second, squinting just a bit. She appears to be engaged in active thought, something I had not seen from the Aussies yet. I think she's trying to work out which insults to hurl at us to convince us to come out.

You can't pike on us tonight!

How dare you fucking pike?!?

Pikey McPikerson!!

All of these are very real possibilities.

"Wait one second," Nico says, ducking back into her room.

She comes back with an enormous plastic bag of prescription-strength medicine. Along with the usual suspects of Tylenol and Advil are some potent allergy medications, antibiotics, and upset stomach pills. For a moment, I feel like we've stumbled onto some Australian drug smuggling ring, which would explain the happiness and the penchant for drink, but I dismiss that explanation as somewhat too cynical.

"Here, you should try some of this," she says, handing Cassie some incredibly strong allergy pills that most people don't exactly come by easily, especially not in a foreign country halfway around the world when you've been on the road for six months.

"Take one of these," Nico says. "And you can keep the rest. Don't worry, I have tons more."

Cassie rotates the pills in her hand. She hesitates for a moment. "How do you have all these medicines?"

"Oh, we're all doctors."

Something clicks in this moment. Here I am, on a vacation that's barely longer than a week, trying to cram in a month's worth of family visits, trips, tourist attractions, and relaxation. I hopped on a flight right after I got off work last Monday, and I will get back to work a few hours before the morning meeting on Thursday. I will return more exhausted than when I left. Up until ten seconds ago, that was the only way I knew how to travel. In my six years working in television news, I never had more than two weeks off, and I worked every single holiday. I knew people took gap years, but I always thought that was only for college students.

Yet these three Aussies are having the time of their lives, and they have very serious and very demanding careers back home. I was never willing to accept or explore the idea that I could travel long-term. I blindly believed that my trips were limited to one- or two-week excursions, racing to a destination, working as hard as possible to squeeze in as much fun as possible, then racing home to get back to my job. And I believed that because everyone else seemed to believe it.

In pursuing the American Dream, we had not dreamed. A split-level house, 1.7 kids, a suburban school. I certainly had a fun job and was enjoying the daily grind that comprises, then defines, a person's daily existence, and I could've kept doing it. Nobody would've questioned me. Except me. I found a glaring contradiction in the midst of my routine: in making a living, I had failed to make a life. The nine-to-five determined the five-to-nine, when it should be the other way around, not just for us, but for everyone.

The last ten years had followed a predictable path from which I had barely strayed. High school to college to grad school to first job to second job . . . Sure, I tried to make my life a little less formulaic. But it still seemed very by-the-book. Only it was a book I had read too many times.

Some people seek nothing more than a quiet, simple life with annual vacations to Florida or California or some other beach destination, and there's absolutely nothing wrong with that if that's what you want. But that's not for me. And not for Cassie. The world is too big, and we had seen too little of it.

I look back on this moment as the genesis of our journey. Without those Australians, I would never have gotten the idea to travel the world, and even if I had had the idea, I certainly would've dismissed it as impossible. It would take me another two years to plan my trip with Cassie, who would by then be my wife despite the objections of certain members of my extended family. But in that short exchange on a random night in Jerusalem, I find inspiration.

And if this moment is inspiration, ten months later I find urgency.

Chapter 2

April 17, 2012
39°57'01.5"N 75°10'02.6"W
Philadelphia, PA, USA

The company at lunch is better than the food. I eat out with one of my best friends, Josh, on a random Tuesday in Philadelphia's Center City. We choose a place that looks decent and sit outside on a beautiful April afternoon. The meal isn't good enough to remember, and the conversation covers work, life, and my upcoming wedding, still five months away. All very normal stuff for us, and I have no reason to believe this week, or even this day, will be any different.

Josh has to work tonight, but my work schedule gives me Tuesdays and Wednesdays off. We go our separate ways, and I am sure I will meet him for a drink near our office on Wednesday night. He doesn't drink, instead opting to smoke an abundance of cigarettes, one pack a day, which sounds awful until you realize he used to smoke two packs a day, making for a commendable 50 percent improvement. One pack suddenly sounds like a good deal! But he hasn't had a drink in five years, so he sips soda while I take care of the beer.

Twenty-four hours later, our mutual friends blow up my phone with texts and calls.

Brigid: "What happened to Josh? Is he okay?"
Bill: "Is he in the hospital?"
Jen: "Have you seen him today?"
Brigid/Bill/Jen: "Did he really have a stroke?"

If there were coffee in my mouth, I would have spit it out. But there is no coffee, so I choke on air.

"Wait, what?! A stroke?"

"Yeah, his mom posted on Facebook that he had a stroke."

I had nothing to do all day, so checking my email and Facebook were not top priorities. I had been content to relax and play the old-school Sega Genesis that, combined with my original Nintendo Entertainment System, make up the only video games I am willing to own and play. Now I have a very pressing need to figure out what the hell is going on.

"Okay, let me see what I can find out. I'll let you know."

There's no way, I think. Josh is thirty-one years old, an age that I am quite confident is far too young for a stroke, not that I really know anything about medicine or neuroscience. But I'm a reporter, and I have a reporter's intuition. Now that intuition, which often functions like an encyclopedia of overly confident guesswork, assures me this is true.

Work confirms Josh is out. His father had called to let them know he wouldn't be in. Josh hasn't called out sick since he started work two years ago, with the exception of one day a couple of weeks ago when he, in fact, wasn't sick. We had spent the whole day hanging out.

Very quickly, it becomes obvious that whatever has happened is pretty damn serious. Josh hates hospitals as much as I hate nursing homes, having watched my grandmother die in one, so he wouldn't allow anyone to take him there unless it were absolutely dire. Still, I can't believe it's a stroke.

I'm at the hospital fifteen minutes later, where I meet my assistant news director, John, who comes over immediately. The hospital is five blocks from my apartment, and at that particular moment, I have no idea how many times I will be making that walk over the next few months.

John is as perplexed as I am. "They're running tests," he says, his brow furrowing in concern above his horn-rimmed glasses.

"Was it really a stroke?"

"Yes."

I call our friend Jen and immediately tell her to get in the car. Josh needs to see her. More importantly, Josh needs her by his side, and she has a three-hour drive from Salisbury. They aren't dating, but they've been great friends for a long time, and they are both integral parts of each other's support system. Josh will need all the support he can get, tonight and every night for a long time.

When I am finally allowed to see Josh, everything hits home. He has a breathing tube in his throat, an IV in his arm, a catheter where catheters go (which the nurse tells me about), and enough monitoring equipment to let out a steady symphony of bings and beeps. It isn't quite Beethoven, but if it's helping, I don't care what it sounds like.

Josh is in and out of a morphine-induced sleep. A white hospital sheet covers his body. His face is swollen from the bleeding, and when the throbbing in his head becomes too much to handle, he arches his whole back, clenches every muscle in his arms and hands, and grunts in excruciating pain. It is awful to watch, but by Josh's side, I watch it again and again. I notice he always twists to his right when the pain gets really bad, and I notice that his right leg isn't moving. The stroke attacked the right side of his body. His has no control over his right leg and barely more than that over his right arm.

The doctor brings over a twisted piece of metal that looks almost like a tuning fork and uses it to test Josh's nerves and sense of touch. His left foot and hand respond quickly. His right hand responds, but only after the doctor puts pressure on his palm. His right leg feels next to nothing. The doctor has to use almost all of her strength to dig the instrument into the bottom of Josh's foot before he reacts.

Among Josh, the doctor, and the nurse, we begin to learn what happened.

Josh is showering before his night shift at work, blasting "Tiny Dancer" by Elton John on his iPhone.

Josh loves the classics—he is a huge Beatles fan—and he always props up his iPhone on the shelf near his shower so he can listen to music as he goes through his daily routine to get ready for work. Today, his choice is Elton John.

He has already powered through "Levon" when "Tiny Dancer" comes on. Elton John's song about the stylish, sexy women of 1970s California is building toward its first chorus two and a half minutes into the song. Josh adds his own off-key harmony to John's stirring vocals.

The stroke hits mid-lyric and levels Josh with the force of a gunshot to the temple. He hits the floor a second later. He is able to force himself to his feet. It will be the last time Josh stands up straight for weeks.

Josh steps out of the shower and collapses again. His right leg isn't responding. He tries to dial 911, but his motor skills are deteriorating too quickly, and he has already forgotten his passcode.

Thankfully, some programmer at Apple decided to add an emergency call feature to the iPhone that doesn't require you to log in. That small feature saves Josh's life. He can't say much, but he repeats his address and says he had a stroke. And he says this over and over again.

Two thoughts cross Josh's mind in the moments before his world goes dark. First, these may be his final minutes on earth. And second, in what could potentially be his final minutes, he is soaking wet, stark naked, and blasting Elton John as loud as his iPhone speakers will allow. This is going to make for one hell of a story for the paramedics. Then it's lights out. He doesn't remember anything else from April 2012.

The paramedics break down the door and rush him to the hospital. I arrive two hours later, when I finally get word of what happened.

We wait for hours, then we wait some more. Answers aren't exactly easy to find here. And I don't mean they're not easy to find in this hospital. I mean answers aren't easy to come by when you're dealing with brain injuries. For every question we ask, and there are many in those first days, we receive a series of answers that each include some degree of guesswork.

The doctor shows us the first CT scans of the stroke. Josh bled 55 to 65 cc's in his brain; 100 cc is the point of no return; doctors say it's nearly impossible for a patient to survive after that. Josh came dangerously close.

"The next twenty-four hours are critical," the neurosurgeon says, stating the obvious. What he doesn't say is that the twenty-four hours after that are critical, and the twenty-four hours after that, and so on and so forth. There is no chance to relax in these first few days, and I am by Josh's bedside as much as work will allow.

I have never believed life has any inclination to be fair. But this— this occurrence, this event, this medical phenomenon—seems way too far over to the other side of the spectrum to be possible. Josh is a veteran, a bronze star recipient, a hero for his service, some might say. A son, a brother, a cousin, an uncle. Above all else, he is a good person (his falsely calling out sick and a few other minor infractions notwithstanding). And here he is, teetering on the precipice of this delicate edge we call life. The slightest push in one direction, and he will be fine. The slightest push in the other . . .

There are signs of hope, and some come almost immediately. I try to make some jokes to lighten the mood a bit when friends come to visit on the first night.

"At least we have conclusive proof that Josh has a brain."

Josh opens his eyes and looks right at me. He is with us, and so is his sense of humor.

Jen arrives shortly before midnight. We stay at Josh's side until 6 a.m., politely ignoring the nurse's insistence that visiting hours are over until we realize that even we have to sleep at some point, and that the waiting room with its off-white fluorescent lighting and poorly padded chairs will not suffice for either of us. Nurses check with Josh every hour, making sure his condition doesn't worsen. He is not allowed to get any real sleep, and this irritates him almost as much as the catheter securely taped to his dick.

When they remove the breathing tube from Josh's throat, they begin asking him questions to check his grasp on reality.

"What's your name?"

"Josh Crompton."

"Where do you live?"

"Philadelphia."

"What year is it?" asks the nurse.

Josh's eyes move under his closed eyelids. "1974." And then, realizing he may be ever so slightly off, he says, "Don't you fucking judge me." Josh is back. I can't help but smile.

Josh doesn't remember much of those first two weeks; he is so loaded up with painkillers. It's probably best that he forgot them. But he doesn't even remember saying his signature line, which he repeats every time I see him.

I enter, squeeze his right hand, and ask, "Hey brother, how's it going?"

Josh murmurs a few words, then gets really pissed off and shouts, "And I can't get any God damn answers around here," before slamming his left fist into the pillow for added emphasis. He always pauses between *God* and *damn*, to let the Almighty know this question is directed partly at the nursing staff and partly at Him. And he *always* slams his left fist into the pillow.

Cassie and I laugh every time we hear it, and it becomes our catch phrase when we visit Josh. We all enjoy yelling, "Can you get any God damn answers around here?" so we can trigger Josh's inevitable response.

"I can't get any God damn answers around here," he screams, as if it's the first time he's saying it. Little do I know it *is* the first time he's saying it, no matter how many times he's said it before. Between the blood in his brain and the painkillers in his system, his short-term memory is shot. He never remembers saying his signature line, not while he's in the hospital, and not after he leaves.

Josh's doctors predict he won't walk again. As a way of giving them the middle finger, Josh starts walking soon after he gets to rehab. His right ankle is still shaky, but he is doing great. And he stops smoking.

Somewhere in the middle of all this—camped by Josh's bedside at night, listening to the hum of the medical machinery surrounding me, or watching Josh try to walk as he balances on a shopping cart, or seeing Josh struggle as he tries to make basic connections in an occupational therapy workbook—I can't help but think about how fragile and fleeting life can be.

One afternoon we're eating lunch together. The next afternoon, Josh is in the hospital struggling to survive. We've been great friends ever since 2006, when he walked into my bureau at WBOC in Dover, Delaware, and handed me his résumé. I remember how much he reeked of smoke, and how much his résumé reeked of smoke, and how much I had never realized that a single piece of paper could actually reek that much of anything without the generous application of scratch-and-sniff stickers. We became friends almost immediately, even living together for a year before I moved to a new job. We shared an apartment and, before he stopped drinking, more than a few beers together. And now, though our friendship hasn't changed at all, our lives have changed dramatically.

I come to one conclusion. It is time to travel.

I have no way of knowing right now how much my life will parallel Josh's, that once we begin our adventure, I will be only months away from my own life-threatening medical trauma. My life will, much like Josh's at this particular moment, descend into medical chaos—a diagnosis that will come out of nowhere and affect every moment of my existence. Only in my case, it happens halfway around the world.

Cassie and I get married a few months later. Josh asks to speak at our wedding, and his speech brings me to tears. I still can't watch the video of the speech without crying. All he does is say thank you, yet it's one of the most emotional speeches I've ever heard.

After the wedding, Cassie and I began planning the trip. The future contains only promise, and we revel in our own sense of temporary immortality.

Chapter 3

August 29, 2013
39°56'45.1"N 75°16'16.9"W
Lansdowne, PA, USA

My last day at work passes with the same fluid routine as the approximately 2,085 other days of work I have clocked over the last eight years. I go to the morning meeting, I am assigned a story, I have six hours to put my story together, I am live on-air during the 5 p.m. or 6 p.m. news. Often both.

In the back of my mind, I keep on standby the two lines I must have ready at all times. "Live in (today's location), Oren Liebermann, CBS 3 Eyewitness News" and "I'm sorry, we're experiencing technical difficulties at this moment." One I use all the time; the other is always there in case the proverbial shit meets the whirling fan in the midst of a live broadcast, which happens more often than it should, at least according to the latest poll of viral YouTube videos.

As a television news reporter, my days become a matter of rote repetition—that is, barring any severe weather. The tiniest whiff of a thunderstorm and we are wall-to-wall with breaking weather coverage. If a branch falls down and blocks even the smallest sliver of a remote dirt road, we find that branch, zoom in tight to make it look enormous, and find someone nearby who says the thunder sounded like a freight train. After a few years in news, even weather becomes a simple function of reiteration.

"I'm standing here at the corner of (fill in street names), where it's been raining since (fill in time). Neighbors here lost power at (fill in another time). We've seen flooded streets along the way, like (fill in more street names). The rain has turned roads into rivers, and the wind has really kicked up these last couple of hours."

Then my station will cut to another reporter who says the same thing in different words, since the weather at point A is, by meteorological rules and empirical evidence, almost the exact same weather at a point B, which is less than twenty miles from point A. String together a few of these reporters and you suddenly have a newscast. Then wait fifteen minutes, go back to the first reporter who is standing in weather that looks awfully similar to the weather from fifteen minutes ago, and repeat the cycle.

Most days, especially in Philadelphia, we cover crime. Or we cover the effects of crime, or someone's attempt to fix the city's crime problem, or the mayor's latest initiative to fight crime, or how much crime has gone up since the mayor's latest initiative to fight it. I try to make my stories more personal, but even crime begins to feel like déjà vu.

"(Mother's name) will never see her son again. (Son's name) was killed when police say someone shot the (fill in age)-year-old in the back at (fill in time)."

On this day though, there is no crime, or at least no major violent crime, which means it's one of three or four good days a year in the Philly metro. Just someone stealing football supplies from Lansdowne County's Penn Wood High School locker room a few months after another student—although possibly the same student—torched the same school before finals. My cameraman and I knock out quick interviews with the coach and assistant coach, grab a statement from police, shoot a few quick shots of the football field, and call it a day.

I've enjoyed nearly every moment of my three years here. Even if TV news is in trouble as a business, in large part because of mobile and the Web, it is one hell of a fun industry to work in. No two days are alike. Though the weeks share a cognitive similarity and my mind goes through the same process every time I write a script, each day is at least geographically and socially different. I see new places and meet new people all the time.

I'm generally nowhere near my bosses, and I get along great with all the cameramen, which is essential considering how much time we spend together in live trucks and how much beer we drink both on and off the clock.

We've been through Hurricane Irene, Superstorm Sandy, the Jerry Sandusky sex scandal, the Catholic Church sex scandal, the Basement of Horrors sex scandal, and hundreds of other stories—a disturbing number of them sex scandals, but not nearly as many as the number of shootings—that I don't particularly care to remember. Some stories are easy to put together, others are a royal pain in the ass.

My goal every day is the same: enjoy lunch. During summer, my goal is slightly more complex. Do a story at the beach . . . and enjoy lunch. Most days, I am successful at least on the latter part.

Initially, I signed on for two years, then re-upped for one more year when Cassie landed a great promotion at her job and we decided to hold off on traveling for a year so we could save more money. After three years in Philly, I can tell you the best place to get a sandwich (Koch's Deli), the best place to get a drink (Prohibition Taproom), the best ice cream (Franklin Fountain), and all sorts of other superlative locations in the City of Brotherly Love. Philadelphia has stopped feeling like a location and started feeling like home. Reporting is no longer my job. It is my career.

I fell into TV news in much the same way dinosaurs fell into vast pits of hot tar. It was unintentional and, once the process began, inescapable. All I wanted to be growing up was a pilot. Specifically a fighter pilot, though any type of pilot would have been just fine. My dad would have none of it, and he sent me to study business in college. Seems like a wise move, right? A young Jewish boy goes into business. What could *possibly* go wrong?!

In 2001, I was watching the NBA playoffs, having just discovered that sports can be fun to both watch and play. (You'll have to forgive me. I was on the debate team in high school, so sports weren't exactly my thing. I went to debate camp—twice.) I instantly decided that I was a diehard Sacramento Kings fan and that I hated the Lakers, never mind that I had never been to LA or Sacramento and had only stepped foot on Californian soil once.

Some time later, while watching a Kings game, I had the epiphany that inadvertently set my life on a path it would follow for the next decade. I say epiphany only to give this moment some weight. In reality, I just had a hunch of something that sounded like fun, and I decided to follow the thought—one that might be most accurately described as a brain fart—to its logical conclusion.

My epiphany was that I was going to do the radio play-by-play for the Sacramento Kings. No one was going to talk me out of this. It was my destiny. Except for one problem: I had no idea how to go about doing the play-by-play for the Sacramento Kings, let alone any sports team in any sport.

I called up an FM station back home, WRAT 95.9 The Rat, and landed a summer internship in the promotions department. My job description was basically to wear a station T-shirt and hit on girls, which was pretty difficult for me since I was painfully shy then. Halfway through the summer, one of the DJs, Steve Hook, sat me down while we were both working at a Lakewood Blueclaws game. The afternoon broadcast had just wrapped up, and he was sitting in the open door of our truck smoking a cigarette, probably after consuming between one and six beers since the station was running a promo series with the recently released Sam Adams Light.

"What the hell are you doing here, kid?" I'm not sure he knew my name then (or now). He also had no idea how much this short conversation would affect my life.

I summoned up all the courage I could find and said in my most manly voice, "I'm going to do the play-by-play for the Sacramento Kings." I'm sure it sounded as idiotic then as it does in your head now.

"Hmm." He paused. "Then here's what ya do." His advice came between puffs of cigarettes, as if even the shortest respite from vaporized nicotine would take the signature rasp out of his voice. "Go back to school. Call up the local AM station and do whatever it takes to get on-air. Whatever ya gotta do." His deep, gravelly voice was perfect for radio, and I can still hear him saying those words. True to my word, I went back to my third year of college at the University of Virginia and called up WINA 1070 AM in Charlottesville, VA. I showed up for my interview in a suit, and I have never been more overdressed. I was lucky. The sports director wanted to expand the station's sports coverage, and he was looking for free labor, which I was more than happy to provide.

"We'll bring you along slowly," he said. "First, we'll have you shadow our sports guys as they go out on stories, then you'll voice your own pieces that don't air, and eventually, you'll do your own stories. You'll be ready in a few months. Probably three."

Steve Hook was right. I was on my way. I didn't quite know where I was headed, but I was definitely going there.

Five days later, my sports director called me.

"Do you want to do live updates from our high school football show?" My training was over before it began. I would give a pregame, halftime, and postgame update from high school football games. To most people, especially those who attended high school football games or paid any attention to major American sports leagues, this wouldn't have been a big challenge. Except I did neither of those. I never went to a single Ocean Township High School Spartans football game and I never paid any attention to the NHL, MLB, NASCAR, MLS, NFL, or any other league, with the recent exception of the NBA.

I was terrified, but I wasn't going to pass up the opportunity. I had no idea whether I would succeed or crash and burn, but it was definitely going to be one of those extremes. There would be no middle ground here.

That game on a random Friday night was the first time I was ever on-air. It was the beginning of what would become my career. And it was absolutely dreadful. I mean God-awful in the truest sense of the Lord's name. If the Almighty had tuned into that particular broadcast, he probably would've struck me down with a lightning bolt or sent Moses to afflict me with plagues 1, 3, 5 to 7 inclusive, and 9.

Yet, for some unfathomable reason, I was asked to do it again the next week. Somehow, I had found a way to crash and burn while succeeding.

For the next two years, I covered all sorts of high school and college sports. If you've ever wondered what kind of radio wannabe does the high school junior varsity girls' field hockey updates, you have your answer. I worked my way up to covering college football and basketball, which, at least to me, felt like the big leagues. I decided it was time to get better. I signed up for graduate school at Syracuse University, the academic mecca of broadcast journalism. I was determined to follow in the footsteps of Bob Costas, Mike Tirico, and Kevin Maher. And that lasted for all of one week.

At the time, Syracuse's program focused on news. They viewed sports as a side project that some of the men in the program pursued in their spare time. On the first day of class, my professor gave me a basic news test. I failed. Miserably. I couldn't even name the three network anchors, who were Dan Rather, Peter Jennings, and Tom Brokaw. But my professor was not one to sugarcoat anything.

"You don't want to do sports radio. You don't know shit about sports, and you don't want to work in radio."

"So what should I do?"

"You're going to do TV news."

"But why? I don't know anything about TV or news."

"You'll figure it out."

That's all it took. I abandoned the epiphany I had in college and focused on TV news. At a Syracuse recruiting day, a small station from Salisbury, Maryland, came up to meet some of the prospective reporters. I signed up for the first interview spot of the morning, and after a few trips to Salisbury to meet the managers and see the newsroom, I landed my first job in TV news.

I spent two years at my first job, working the night shift out of the bureau in Dover, Delaware, a city that sextuples in size during NASCAR races. I was only two hours south of the upper middle class suburban town where I grew up, yet I felt like I was somewhere in the middle of Alabama, especially when hordes of race fans invaded the miniscule metropolis with their cases of Miller Lite and wads of chewing tobacco. Josh was one of the cameramen here—his stroke would come years later, long after we left the station.

Two significant things happened at my first job. First, I earned my pilot's license on March 14, 2007. I had wanted to be a pilot for as long as I could remember. I built model airplanes as a kid and read every book I could about flying. I knew what every instrument in a cockpit did long before I was ever allowed to climb into one. Although I consider this to be one of the most important days of my life, it is almost completely irrelevant to the rest of this story. Almost.

The second significant thing that happened in Dover was that I was kicked out of my job. I asked my managers if I could get out of my two-year contract early so I could find my next job and move up in the world, since I aspired to greater heights than making $26,000 in Delaware, a state so insignificant it couldn't come up with anything more recent than "The First State" to put on its license plates (they had to go back to the signing of the Declaration of Independence to find a noteworthy event in the state's history). My managers agreed to let me go. I was free to leave as soon as I found my second job. But less than a month later they announced a new hire.

Some girl named Cassandra Kramer. She was a Temple University graduate. And she would work the night shift at Dover. They had hired my
replacement.

I was being forced out.

I was furious. I was so pissed off that day I forgot my camera on a shoot
and had to go back to the station to get it. I vowed I would never do anything to help this new reporter. She could learn for herself how to deal with
the managers, how to find stories, how to report breaking news, who she
had to know, and all of the other nuances and tricks that make a reporter's
job easier. She was dead to me.

We got married five years later.

One month after Cassie took over my shift at my first station, I took my
second job in Norfolk, Virginia. It was the perfect place to be for an eager
young reporter. We had great cameramen, awesome managers, and it was a
fun city. I spent three years there before it was time to move on.

By this time, Cassie had left TV news and was finishing up her graduate
degree at the University of Delaware. She had had a passion for teaching
English as a second language ever since she spent a summer in Ecuador
while in college, and that's what she studied for her master's degree. She
landed a job teaching in Philadelphia, and thanks to Josh's help (he was, by
now, working on the assignment desk at the CBS affiliate in Philly), I got a
job reporting there. Cassie and I moved in together, and I proposed on the
morning of her graduation, having called in sick to ensure that I wouldn't be
late to the commencement ceremonies. I wish I had some great, romantic
story of how I proposed or a YouTube video that went viral to which I could
point you, but I just wrapped the ring as her graduation gift and gave it to
her over breakfast. Nothing goes together like coffee and diamonds.

After two years in Philadelphia, we wed near her parents' home in
Macungie, a town that was virtually unknown until a local couple stole a
cop car in New Jersey a few months before our wedding, led a wild police
chase across the Ben Franklin Bridge into Pennsylvania, stole another cop
car while police were busy stopping the first cop car, led a second wild
police chase, and finally got caught.

Right before our wedding, I signed a one-year extension in Philadelphia. Cassie and I weren't yet sure if we were traveling, but we were planning our trip and saving for it as if it were a sure thing.

We stopped going out to eat, stopped buying new clothes, stopped going on weekend trips, and stopped spending money on anything we considered luxurious or unnecessary. We even scaled back on our wine consumption.

By April 2013, we were committed. Over the next few months, we sold off as much of our furniture as we could. We put her car up for sale and donated my car, since there was no way anyone would pay money for a 2001 Toyota Camry with 260,000 miles on it and an eclectic array of dings and scratches. As we sold everything we deemed unnecessary, we bought all sorts of things that were suddenly very necessary in the process of trading one life for another. We swapped our living room for a backpack, our cars for hiking shoes, our kitchen for a water filtration bottle, our suits for dry-fit shirts and pants, and our medicine cabinet for a portable first-aid kit. We drastically downsized our lives. In the end, everything we could still call our own fit into a seven-by-ten storage space, and there was plenty of room to spare.

We were ready for our trip. We banked $17,000 from our wedding and $23,000 more over the year, leaving us a tidy $40,000 in our savings account. I just had to get through the last few months of work. Some live shots, a bit of breaking news, a smattering of crime stories, and storms to cover. No big deal.

Then I nearly forced us to cancel the trip.

Early in the summer, I signed up for an ultimate frisbee league with Cassie's brother. I've played ultimate frisbee ever since high school, progressing from friendly pick-up games to organized tournaments. I figured I would play one last league to get in shape for the trip.

Halfway through our first game, my team was on defense, trailing 5–4, when the guy I was covering ran deep. He sprinted straight for the end zone, and I was right behind him. The frisbee went up. It was coming in behind me and to my right. I jumped and twisted in midair to intercept the frisbee or at least knock it out of the air, when I realized I had mistimed the jump. I knew instantly the disc would sail about a foot beyond my reach, and my guy would score. Instead of paying attention to the ground toward which I was now rapidly accelerating with the usual 9.8 meters per second squared that gravity exerts on a falling object, I focused on the disc and the player I was chasing.

My right foot touched the ground first, and I was blinded with pain. I knew what happened in the brief but interminable instant before I collapsed on the field. I had blown out my ACL. The sickening snap, the shock of pain, the unnatural twist. It couldn't be anything else. A player on my team fifteen feet away from me heard the tear, almost like a cartoonish pop. I had never torn my ACL before, but I'd heard enough people describe it to be fairly certain that's what happened.

My first thought was, "Holy shit, this hurts." My second thought was, "Holy shit, I might've just ruined our trip."

An ambulance took me to the Hospital of the University of Pennsylvania, covering the half-mile in forty-five minutes, horns blaring and lights flashing the entire way. At the hospital, a resident had me put weight on my right leg. When she saw I could stand on one foot, she concluded that I hadn't torn my ACL.

"It looks like you just sprained it," she said.

She was wrong and I knew it, but I didn't argue. That was a mistake. Because she didn't approve an MRI on the spot, it took me two weeks of yelling at my insurance company to have one approved. The MRI confirmed what I already knew. I had torn my right ACL. And I needed surgery, followed by months of physical therapy. Unlike other parts of the body, the ACL can't heal itself. A torn anterior cruciate ligament will stay forever torn unless it is surgically repaired. You can forgo surgery and live without an ACL, but then your list of allowable athletic activities shrinks dramatically since the ACL is the major stabilizing ligament in the knee. No, I would need to go under the knife.

You generally have three options for a new ACL tendon. You can have a piece of your patella tendon cut from the front of your knee and attached to your ACL. You can use a piece of your hamstring tendon from the back of your leg. Or you can go with option three. You can have an Achilles tendon taken out of the ankle of a cadaver and put into your knee as your brand new, sort-of-used ACL. I chose option three. My new ACL came from a dead guy I didn't know but to whom I am eternally grateful. If the zombie apocalypse ever comes, I consider myself immunized since I am one percent undead.

I thought tearing my ACL would be the great medical challenge of our trip. Man, was I wrong.

Between physical therapy and all the doctor's appointments, I missed most of my last three months at work. I was in a locked leg brace for six weeks, an unlocked brace for one more week, and had to learn to walk normally again after that.

I asked my doctor and my physical therapist if I could still travel. They both gave the same answer.

"Yes, but no jogging, no jumping, no running, no sports, no doing anything but walking wherever you have to go."

Okay, I thought. Simple enough. I could manage that.

I have only five weeks of work left when I'm finally able to return, and I have a severe case of professional senioritis. I do everything I can to avoid major stories, volunteering for light fluff to cover.

In my eight years in the industry, I have seen more dead bodies than I care to remember, talked to more grieving mothers than I can count, knocked on enough suspects' doors to always feel unsafe, been to enough crime scenes to believe the world really can be a bad place, and stood in enough thunderstorms and hurricanes to feel perpetually wet. I even witnessed an execution.

Local news reporters too often make a living off the lowest rungs of society, profiting just a bit more each time someone pulls a knife or a gun and uses it to add a little more chaos to this world. I am more than happy to step away from that, even if it means emptying my savings account and starting over when I get back.

So, it is no surprise to me when my final story in Philadelphia is about someone stealing football supplies from a high school. At least it's easy, and we find all of the elements we need within a few minutes of showing up.

Many of my closest friends at work plan to join me in a few hours for a drink at the bar we all use as the post-shift pub of choice for consumption of alcohol. I pack up my final few belongings—not much considering how little time I spent at my desk—and make my way to the exit.

I look back one last time at the doors I have walked through every day of my professional life for the last three years. I will certainly remember this place, and, for a brief moment, I think it will remember me too. Then I look at the video monitor that hangs by the entrance.

It says, "Bon Voyage, Owen!"

Chapter 4

September 15, 2013
52°45'01"N 35°30'58"W
Charlie-Gibbs Fracture Zone, North Atlantic Ocean

Any well-thought-out plan for the first day of our trip, factoring in the overnight flight, the early morning landing, the physical rigors of walking around a city and sightseeing all day, and the meeting of our host at night, would mandate that I be asleep right now. But then again, any well-thought-out plan for my greater adult life would mandate that I not quit my job to travel the world with my wife for a year with no prospects for professional employment upon our return, so I think such machinations in general can be liberally ignored and safely discarded, no matter their scope.

We are halfway into the first flight of our trip, US Airways Flight 718, departing from Philadelphia International Airport at 1615; arriving at Roma Fiumicino Airport at 0850, currently 35,000 feet above the Atlantic Ocean. A quick check of the GPS on the nine-inch screen in front of me—or whatever the metric equivalent is since we're headed toward Europe—shows a cartoonishly large airplane.

The nose of the plane is somewhere south of Greenland while the tail of the airplane is still over Massachusetts. Average that out and we must be nowhere near our destination. If they zoomed out any more, it would show a giant plane covering all of North America.

We are one airline meal away from Italy. A hermetically sealed, roughly twelve-by-eight-inch container of yogurt, cheese, water, mixed fruit, and a vegetable du jour separates us from Rome. We savor every bite, knowing that this four-course meal—five if you count the

water—will be our most luxurious feast for a while. From the very beginning, we planned on small snacks from grocery stores and half-sandwiches
from corner bodegas to get us through the trip, so we try to enjoy every
morsel of vacuum-packed US Airways goodness while ignoring the inevitable staleness that inherently comes with anything served six miles above
sea level. With each minute, more of my neighboring passengers turn off
their lights—it's getting to be evening in Philadelphia as our plane inches
toward dawn in Rome.

Meanwhile, I'm sitting here listening to Walk off the Earth on my iPod
and trying to figure out how few hours of sleep I need to get through my
first day and night in Rome. Regardless of what the correct answer is, I
suspect we're about to find out how well two hours will suffice. My internal
calculus notifies me that, on multiple occasions, I have stayed up many
more consecutive hours with far more complex and unquantifiable variables
mixed into the equation. Of course, all of those occasions were in college,
which, to my ever-growing dismay, was nearly a decade ago. But all of that
is currently and forevermore irrelevant.

Even now, halfway through our first flight, it's impossible to comprehend our trip. There is nothing certain ahead of us. Plans change as quickly
as they are made, and one unforeseen event can alter our journey dramatically. It doesn't make us nervous; it excites us—that sense of the unknown
and the stimulus of adventure hidden within each day.

Today is almost exactly our one-year anniversary. I say "almost" because
it is officially six days after the anniversary. Our goal was to leave on September 9, but we postponed our departure to celebrate the Jewish high
holidays with my family. Yom Kippur ended last night. Spiritually cleansed
and hungry as hell, we broke the fast at my brother's home in northern New
Jersey, bade farewell to my family, and spent the night with Cassie's parents
in Allentown, Pennsylvania.

Our final day in the US is a blur. We knock out our last few tasks in
the morning, pack our final few belongings into our backpacks, and head
for Philly. By 1:30 in the afternoon, we're at Molly's Philly apartment in
Brewerytown, dropping off our cats, who are so shell-shocked by the
new place they hardly notice we're gone. Molly is Cassie's best friend
and maid of honor who volunteered to care for our two rescue cats in our
absence. There's Ria, our tan female cat, and her black cat brother, Inigo,

named after Inigo Montoya from *The Princess Bride*. Cassie named Ria; I named Inigo.

A final lunch with friends consists of hot wings and a turkey burger, washed down with a Bloody Mary and a champagne toast to our health and safe travels. Then to the airport and a final farewell to Cassie's parents. Cassie's mom snaps one last picture of us as we hoist our backpacks and head for check-in.

Cassie's dad is smiling. "You should remember this moment. It's the most you're ever gonna weigh!"

Neither of us know how true those words will become in a few months. For now, we enjoy the moment, short though it is.

We breeze through security, always a pleasant surprise when the TSA is running things. Boarding is painfully slow, but we grab our seats early, and I begin the notes that will eventually form this book.

There is a moment of calm on board before the floodgates open. Suddenly, people stream down both aisles on our Airbus A330. The quiet is gone. What's left in its wake is a conglomeration of human faces, smells, and emotions that are the natural consequence of 291 people shoved into a pressurized aluminum tube for eight hours. There is no escape, especially not through the overweight passenger to my right who has sandwiched me into seat 23E. There is denial first, then resignation, and finally acceptance.

I find myself canting slightly to my left to maintain my rapidly shrinking personal space. Around me, people are smashing oversized bags into undersized luggage compartments, fiddling with lights and air vents, and generally trying to get comfortable in a space where the population density is 350 times higher than that of the US.

I had imagined what it would be like to see American soil for the last time as our flight from Philly International arches out over New Jersey and then the Atlantic. I would see the light of the cities—first the City of Brotherly Love, then the Big Apple. I would see the crooked line of the Jersey Shore, inching its way north-northeast. And there's my home, or at least an approximation of where my home should be, since we would be nearing our cruising altitude when we passed it.

That, as it turns out, was a pipe dream. Bereft of both the pipe and the necessary herbal ingredients to place within its hollowed out interior, I have only my view from the middle seat. The window shade to my left, with four people and an aisle between us, has already been closed by an elderly woman who seems to be in complete denial of the fact that she is on an airplane that is about to leave the relatively safe confines of Philadelphia, never mind the fact that you're almost always safer *not* being in Philadelphia. The window shade to my right is open, but all I can see past my rotund companion is a section of wing.

To prepare us for our flight to the ancient city of Rome, US Airways has decided to play a loop of outdoor scenes called "HDenvironments." Corporate must have concluded that the best video for this flight is what I'm pretty sure is Yellowstone and Grand Teton National Parks, where Cassie and I recently spent a week on a family vacation. Not that I have any way of incontrovertibly verifying my opinion, but I suspect people heading for Italy have very little fascination with the geysers and bison of Montana and Wyoming.

A quick glance to my right reveals my neighbor, who has a pamphlet on scripture. For him, this trip is probably a pilgrimage. I consider bursting into Hebrew prayers—the Shema, the Kaddish Shalem, the Birkat Hamazon—but he or some other nearby passenger might confuse Hebrew with Arabic, which I feel would be detrimental to the rest of my trip and the likelihood of the TSA ever allowing me on a plane again.

As we start taxiing, the emergency video launches into its cheery instructional spiel. Everyone is always smiling in these, even though they're preparing for a crash landing. We're taxiing for so long I begin to wonder if we're taxiing to Rome.

And that's when the baby behind me, whom I somehow hadn't noticed to this point, erupts. Volcanic bursts and magmatic spittle in newborn Italian. The woman behind Cassie, perhaps the mother of the baby, announces she doesn't like that she can see the wing out the window. I note this down as the dumbest thing I have heard on this flight so far—and we're still taxiing. There's an "Are we there yet?" to my right. Something garbled in Italian at my 8 o'clock. And more of said shrieking baby.

Our journey is under way.

This flight is the first aerial passage of thirteen we already have booked on our itinerary. Philadelphia to Rome to Ethiopia to Kenya back to Ethiopia to Israel to Thailand. Then a bit of land travel through Southeast Asia to Beijing before flying from Beijing to Tokyo to San Francisco to San Salvador to Lima to Santiago to Toronto back to Philadelphia. Arranged in two long run-on sentences like that is probably the best way to get a feel for our trip. It will be extensive, a bit chaotic, and will almost certainly require us to pause somewhere in the middle to catch our breath.

When we started planning a year ago, we looked at major regions we wanted to visit: Europe, Israel, Southeast Asia, and South America. From there, we picked countries within those regions that interested us.

In Europe, we figured we could sneak five countries into ten weeks. Even though Cassie's been to Italy, I've never been, so that was at the top of our list and the country we would start in. We would make our way north and west into southern France and southern Spain—our next two countries—before looping back through Madrid toward Paris. From Paris, we would book a short flight to Ireland, where we would spend two weeks exploring the various pubs in which to drink Guinness and Murphy's Irish Stout, as well as the people with which to drink them. Our last major country in Europe would be Hungary—both Cassie and I have Hungarian blood.

Israel is our next major stop, with a trip to Jordan to see Petra.

Then we leave the Western world to explore Southeast Asia. A flight into Bangkok and three months of trains, buses, and tuk-tuks through Thailand, Cambodia, Laos, and Vietnam. North from Vietnam into China, then east through China to Beijing, and a flight to Tokyo. A quick stop to visit friends in San Francisco and step foot on American soil for the first time in nine months, then to South America, where we would visit Peru, Chile, and Argentina, with possible side trips to Bolivia, Brazil, and Uruguay. And finally, home.

Laid out on paper, it all seemed so simple.

We just needed to find the gentlest way to impart our desires to travel for a year upon my parents, who were, in my opinion, likely to register more than a few complaints against our trip.

What about your jobs? Who will take care of your cats? How will you make money? What about your safety? What about all the holidays and birthdays you will miss? Why travel for so long?

We visited my parents on a random spring weekend and broke the news to them during dinner at the Houlihan's on Rt. 35 near Monmouth Mall. We sat in a booth and ordered variations of the same generic fare that you find at all of the chain restaurants aspiring to be something greater than what they are or will ever be. A waitress had just brought over the stuffed mushrooms ("with herb and garlic and cream cheese") when I decided it was time.

"So, we're thinking of traveling the world for a year." I made it sound like it wasn't a done deal. I would hold off on that bit of information to see how the conversation progressed. Nothing in my thirty years of existence had prepared me for their response.

"Tamar is moving to Kenya."

"Wait, what?!"

Tamar is my sister, ten years older than me. Her husband, Cam, and two young daughters live in a beautiful house in Upper Middle Class Suburbia north of New York City, where she is as protective of her daughters as she was of me and my twin sister growing up. Of all the members of my family, I would vote her "Least Likely to Move to Africa" and "Most Likely to Overuse Hand Sanitizer," if there were such familial balloting.

"Cam got a job in Africa," explained my mom in her thick Israeli accent, "and they're moving to Kenya in July."

Cassie and I looked at each other. This newfound knowledge could mean only one thing.

"Okay, then we'll add Kenya to our list."

My sister had unknowingly made our news much easier for my parents to accept, and the rest of the conversation went fairly smoothly. We laid out our plans, our country list, and our anticipated return date. My parents' biggest concern was the length of the trip. They wanted us to travel for three months or maybe six months, but not twelve.

"But then we come home in the middle of the school year," Cassie pointed out. "If we travel a full year, we come home before next school year, and I can find a job easily."

The rest of my family registered varying degrees of objections and endorsements to our travels. Hadas, my twin sister, was all for it. She and her husband, Jay, had spent five months in Vietnam a few years ago, so they were practically ready to travel with us, if not for their infant son and the financial and medical demands of parenthood, not to mention the custom leatherwork company they had just started. Tamar was excited that she already had her first family visitor and began making preparations posthaste, even though a few months separated us from traveling and her from

Kenya. As expected, she worried about our safety and sent us messages across all forms of digital media about preparations she felt were judicious and precautions she felt were necessary.

My brother Erez, eight years older than me, was the most stringently opposed to our travels. He kept asking the same question, "What will you do for work when you get back?" varying the verbiage ever so slightly each time to make it seem like he was posing a different question. "How will you find a job when you get back?" "What about employment when you get back?" Every question ended in ". . . when you get back?" He asked the same question so many times in so many different ways that I began to wonder if he stayed up late at night writing down ways to phrase what was effectively the same query. To him, it was neither the journey nor the destination that was important. It was the nine-to-five job I would find after I had completed the journey and reached the destination that should be the ultimate achievement of our trip.

When I told him we didn't really care about finding a job after our travels when we hadn't even started them yet, he always said, "All right," in a tone of voice that sounded like he was rolling his eyes, even if his pupils remained stationary. From the very beginning, I had no doubt we would not see him anywhere on our trip.

With a little more finessing and a lot more blind guesswork, we finished our rough itinerary. We didn't need to know every detail of the trip; we needed a vague outline and a list of cities. We would figure out the minutiae on the fly, planning about two weeks ahead on the road. We knew we would have to book some short flights in Europe to get between, say, Ireland and Hungary, but there was no pressing need to worry about that yet. Much to my dismay, Australia and New Zealand were not on our itinerary. Our round-the-world ticket had a cap of 39,000 miles; with the addition of Kenya, the Outback and its neighboring islands would have to wait. At least I thought they were neighboring, until I checked a globe and realized New Zealand wasn't all that close to Australia and was, in fact, more closely aligned with the Pacific Ocean's version of the middle of nowhere. Fortunately, I didn't have to worry about getting there. We booked our flights.

At 8:15 on a Monday morning, we touch down in Rome—thirty-five minutes early—swapping countries, continents, and lifestyles.

We hit the ground running in Rome, almost as if we're using the iner-tia of the airplanes to propel us through the small tasks we have to finish before we can start exploring. Grab a shuttle to the train station. Store our luggage at Roma Termini. Grab a SIM card for our cell phone.

We could take the metro for a quick ride to the Colosseum, but we walk instead, soaking up as much of the Italian culture and language as we can in our first twenty minutes in Rome. We learn two critical words immediately: *grazie* and *Nutella*.

Even from a distance, the size of the Colosseum is breathtaking, espe-cially for something built two thousand years ago. It is as beautiful as it is intricate. Above ground are the arches that support the massive structure and seats. Below ground are the maze-like pathways that led gladiators and animals into battle and, in most cases, death. It's easy to imagine the roaring crowd, cheering on the warriors and thirsting for the mixture of sport and violence that played out on the arena floor.

History radiates from every building and every street in this area. Nearby is Palatine Hill and the Roman Forum, steeped in millennia of antiq-uity. In America, if something is three hundred years old, it's considered historically significant. Here, if it's only three hundred years old, it's junk, not even worth a footnote in Fodor's. The stories of past centuries echo off the walls and cascade down the streets, washing over us in a breathtaking waterfall of history. You don't see history in Rome so much as you feel it surrounding you. You breathe it in with each step as you walk through the capital of the Roman empire. The structures that still stand—the Colos-seum, the Forum—are a testament to the greatness of Caesar's realm and what man could accomplish before the invention of business meetings and paperwork.

By this point, we are exhausted and jet-lagged on our first day of travel. Given our lack of sleep on the flight, we are at a solid twenty-six hours without anything that qualifies as rest. If we had any idea at this moment that we wouldn't sleep for another nine hours, we might simply collapse. But we don't know that, so we keep moving, fueled mostly by adrenaline since we have decided not to splurge yet on our first Italian coffee or gelato.

We take a few back roads to the Pantheon, intentionally avoiding the clogged tourist streets. We get happily lost once or twice and wander around Rome for a bit, drinking in the culture and the coffee. Starbucks, take note: the coffee here puts your eighteen-dollar latte to shame. It's comforting to know that in Rome, you can always find an equally lost English-speaking tourist who can help you find your way. Or you both get lost together, which is just as fun.

Our meandering route takes us through back alleys and narrow pathways, high walls and clogged streets, bringing us to the Pantheon from behind the famed structure. This building holds a special place in my heart, because the Rotunda at my alma mater, the University of Virginia, is based on the Pantheon. But as much as I love UVA, the Jeffersonian imitation doesn't quite compare to the real thing. The beauty of the Pantheon is worth looking at from every angle—outside and inside, close up and far away. The piazza out front is a great place to sit and admire the Pantheon while sharpening your pickpocket avoidance skills.

We visit the Trevi fountain, marveling at both the mythical statues and the seemingly infinite number of people crammed into a noticeably finite space to stare at the mythical statues. We wrap up our day with a walk through some of the famous piazzas here—Popolo, Spagna, Repubblica, and San Pietro—and a look at the Spanish steps, which is apparently the afternoon meeting spot for most of Rome.

Finally, after thirty-one hours without sleep, it's time to meet our couch-surfing host. Our accommodations for the first month on the road rely heavily on couchsurfing, a network of strangers that pairs travelers with hosts. A registered traveler reaches out to a group of similarly registered hosts in a town or city and asks if any have a spare couch or bed for a few nights. Generally, the traveler and the host are complete strangers, and the two read reviews from other users to figure out if the other person is trustworthy. No money is ever exchanged between host and hosted. Instead, the guest will (or at least should) bring some sort of small gift or do a chore for the host.

Knowing that we would couchsurf on our trip, we registered through the website a few months ago and started hosting travelers. In the three or four months before we started our own trip, we hosted six people: a French-Moroccan guy, a Chinese guy, a Dutch girl, a Chinese girl, and an Israeli woman. We thought our open show of hospitality and faith in the rest of humanity—or at least the segment of the rest of humanity that travels internationally—would inspire our friends. In fact, most of them thought we were batshit crazy. They peppered us with a barrage of passive-aggressive questions to try to convince us to cease and desist any and all couchsurfing–related activities.

"So you have strangers sleeping in your house?"

"Do you feel safe?"

"What keeps them from robbing you?"

"What keeps them from *killing* you?"

Those questions aren't totally unreasonable. A quick Web search for "Couchsurfing nightmares" leads to the following top five results: 1) "A Traveler's Nightmare: Couchsurfing in NYC," 2) "Couchsurfing Sucks Couchsurfing Horror Stories," 3) "Madrid—The Worst Couchsurfing Experience in the World," 4) "'Rape' horror of tourist who used couchsurfing website," and 5) "An opportunity or a nightmare? The Truth about Couch Surfing."

But if we were afraid of what might happen when we stepped out of our comfort zone, we would never have gone on this trip in the first place. Every action, with the possible exception of "stay in bed all day with only the minimum number of trips to the kitchen and bathroom," involves a certain amount of risk, and you can find a reason to dismiss something as "too dangerous" or "too risky" if you look hard enough.

In fact, a quick Web search for "chocolate cake nightmares" leads to the following top five results: 1) "Weight Watcher's Nightmare Chocolate Cake recipe," 2) "The Chocolate Cake Nightmare | Hellgirl: Clever Mommy Blog," 3) "Chocolate 'can give you nightmares'" 4) "Does eating CHOCOLATE CAKE and ICE CREAM before going to sleep........?????," and 5) "Clues: A Paranoid Schizophrenic's Detective Story."

We were happy to accept the risk of inviting strangers into our home so we could meet new people, swap stories, and share experiences. In many ways, we had begun our world travels without ever leaving our living room. Most of our couchsurfing guests cooked dinner for us, and a few brought us small gifts, such as an Eiffel Tower keychain from Paris. They showed us pictures of where they grew up, told us what to see in their country, and invited us to stay with their family.

Now, for the first time, we are on the other side of the relationship. Instead of hosting, we are traveling, and we are to meet our host at 8:00 in the evening at Piazza Repubblica.

Gianfranco picks us up in the piazza along with another couchsurfer he is hosting—Louise from France. Gianfranco is somewhere in his late thirties or early forties. He is not too thin and not too tall, but neither is he not too fat and not too short. His hair might once have been described as thick and dark, but it is only a shadow of its former self; he is thinning up top and in front, a few steps ahead of my own mutinous pompadour. He sports a short stubble and a quick smile, and he offers to help Cassie with her backpack and daypack immediately. He welcomes us to Italy and to Rome with only a hint of an Italian accent, making his English very easy to understand.

Louise looks to be in her mid-twenties, a student who finished some degree of education, left her native France, and is now moving to Rome to add another degree of education. She has short cropped hair, and she makes it look great with her thick-rimmed glasses. I would describe her hair and clothing as Euro-chic, even though I have barely any idea what that means (though I suspect those who use the term far more frequently also have barely any idea what it means). I wonder if the similarities between Louise and Cassie—young, attractive, female—help explain why Gianfranco was so willing to host us.

The four of us sandwich ourselves and our luggage into what passes in Europe for a car but in America would barely qualify as a functioning golf cart. We head for Gianfranco's apartment near Castelnuovo—a small town outside of Rome built around a castle. The night is about to begin. Sleep will have to wait.

We pick up pizza on the way to meet Gianfranco's friends, who live way off the beaten path. To be fair, everything looks way off the beaten path when you're speeding along small, unlit roads in a foreign country with a stranger who believes speed limits are more suggestions than enforceable laws. At their place, out comes fresh pasta and beer and weed to go with small rectangles of pizza, which we couldn't help but notice were heretically "sliced" with scissors. We are strangers here but are welcomed as friends. By the end of the night, we are part of la famiglia. We traded in the comforts of home and a living room and a bed. Instead, we have a train and a backpack and a couch. This is our new life. This is our new home.

Gianfranco pulls out a guitar and starts singing. Soon the guitar is passed around the table—anyone who wants can sing and strum. Gianfranco's friend even pulls out a harmonica for accompaniment.

The night progresses into a whirling cyclone of music and friendship. After Gianfranco sings, he recharges with beer and pizza while Louise sings. Gianfranco's friend opts for a slightly different and less nutritious fulfillment, a marijuana joint that's passed around as liberally as the other snacks and libations. We don't smoke—we didn't before and we're not about to start—but especially on the first night of our adventure, it seems so unnecessary. The songs are a mix of Italian hits and English classics, and we sing along when we can. The day is special for so many reasons—our first day of travel, seeing the Colosseum, etc.—and the night is magical.

For just a little bit longer, Cassie and I are able to put off sleep. We are sitting with six people we've never met, and we're all laughing and singing as if we've been friends for years. Language barriers fall away. Nationalities don't matter. We all have one thing in common at this very moment—we're all happy, enjoying every moment in our present company.

When Monday finally turns into Tuesday, we call it a night and head back to Gianfranco's home. We haven't slept in thirty-five hours and are still fighting jetlag. But our first day in Italy is without equal—a day we will never forget, and a night that will always be special to us.

We are asleep before our heads hit the pillow.

Two days later we catch a morning train from Rome and head to Florence, then keep going north along the Ligurian coast. Towns on the Italian countryside fly by in a blur of blue and white train station signs—ALOSSIS, ANDORA, DIANO MARINA—their inhabitants no more aware of our existence than we are of theirs. We call ourselves travel bloggers, which is a fancy term for vagrants.

Sometimes we sleep. Sometimes we write. Sometimes we stare out into the hinterlands of whatever region we're passing through and daydream. Out here, we are on our own plane of existence. Back home, our friends are at work or at home—doing what people normally do in life, or rather what life normally does to people. We miss weddings and baby showers and birthdays, reading about all these events on our Facebook newsfeeds and adding our "Congratulations!" and "Mazel Tovs!" For the big events, we add our "Like," as if another click on the World Wide Web is a decent substitute for us being there.

We live in a state of travel—an imaginary place somewhere between Valhalla and Elysium—where we can pretend time stands still. We don't age on this trip—we experience. Hours and minutes and seconds don't affect us like they do other people, unless they're on a train schedule, in which case they affect us in a very real and concrete way. It would be nice to think we can pick up our lives without interruption when we get back, but that's not the truth. What is? What will we come back to? We race toward that answer with each flight and every train ride, blissfully ignorant of what the future has in store.

Chapter 5

November 13, 2013
49°34'36.0"N 19°50'08.0"E
Spytkowice, Poland

One must glimpse a busload of passengers halfway through a seven-hour trip traversing the Eastern European countryside to fully understand the contorted positions in which the human body can sleep. Our Orangeways bus—nothing like the bright, shiny mass transportation vehicle we had seen online—pulled out of Budapest at 7 a.m., destined for Krakow by early afternoon. The bus is probably half full, and couples split up to spread out and take advantage of empty seats. I imagined sleep would be easy to come by once we got on the highway and were cruising through northern Hungary, Slovakia, and southern Poland. But through an abundance of poor planning, either on the part of our driver or on the part of the local transportation authorities, we never come by any highways.

Zsdrabrweg, as I imagined his name to be (or some other combination of seemingly random letters that always starts with one or more Z's), sticks to back roads the whole way. The countryside is beautiful. Or at least I imagine it would be if we could see any of it. From the moment we leave, the sky is covered in a low, gray overcast of uniform color and opacity and a light, constant drizzle that obscures anything more than a few hundred yards away, sometimes much less. Oftentimes, we drive through valleys that climb so steeply I can't see much more than the road and the ominous gray that we keep driving toward and receding from—always there, yet always slightly out of reach. Even the yellows and greens and reds of autumn seem somehow monochromatic in this atmosphere.

The weather is appropriate, given why we're heading to Krakow. I can't imagine Poland ranks very high on any traveler's "Must See" list for Europe, but I had two requirements when we started planning our journey. One, I have to stop and see my family in Israel, even though we'd been there fairly recently. And two, I have to see Auschwitz. The omnipresent grayness fits the purpose of our visit. Dark and forlorn. Cold and wet. We will find nothing uplifting in Auschwitz—not in the skies above or on the ground below—nor do we expect to.

The Polish countryside (or is it the Slovakian countryside? I didn't see the border crossing) looks much as I had expected it to appear. Vastly empty with sporadic houses along the streets. There is no single design or style that dominates construction, except maybe the liberal use of concrete. Multicolored is not a word that comes to mind. We don't see many people outside, and if not for the smoke drifting upward from some of the chimneys, the few homes we see would look completely deserted. It occurs to me that even the smoke looks like it's trying to escape.

Cassie sits to my right across the aisle, the seats staggered so she's slightly behind me. She is listening to her iPod, probably something uplifting to get her mind off the weather and the purpose of our visit. I prefer to ride in silence, thinking about the visit to Auschwitz and contemplating our surroundings.

Our bus isn't particularly comfortable. A row of heaters runs along the lower edge of the window, eking out a few degrees of warmth if you nestle right up to it. Eighteen inches away in the aisle seat, I sit beyond the range of the heater, where it is at least fifteen degrees colder. Balancing my laptop on my somewhat spread out legs, made necessary by the inability of the seats to accommodate someone taller than five-foot-eight, I can feel the difference in temperature between my left leg—closer to the heater—and my right leg in the passenger bus–equivalent of the Arctic Circle. We are a thousand miles away from any Spanish-speaking country, yet all of our windows say PROHIBIDO FUMAR. Those signs must have been added after the ashtrays in the back of every seat, when some managers finally acknowledged that, yes, smoking may in fact be bad for you.

Yet I know I am infinitely more comfortable than my first relatives to make this journey—the family of my maternal grandmother. They came from a different direction—from Zdunska Wola in central Poland via the Lodz ghetto—but their destination was the same: Auschwitz. They came by train, crammed together in an endless row of cattle cars, seen as no more worthy of life than the previous bovine passengers. When one train ended, another soon took its place. I often wondered why my family didn't try to escape. Now I wonder if I'll have a better sense of that after our visit to Poland.

Although the rain keeps falling, the temperature stays above freezing, holding at about forty-two degrees. We had expected it to be colder— much colder—our knowledge of Eastern European climatology clouded by pictures we had seen of Poland from World War II. It was always snowing in those photos, and somehow, we expected it to always be snowing in Poland, regardless of month or season.

Twenty minutes from our scheduled arrival time, we begin to see blocks of concrete closer together and a bit more frequently. Ah, these must be the suburbs of Krakow. Even the car dealerships look like they are made of concrete, although presumably they were constructed recently enough to be made of something else. I guess the Poles didn't want to break the monotony of their countryside. A bright, colorful billboard advertising four different kinds of chocolate bars—milk chocolate, cherry, caramel, and neon blue—looks completely out of place.

Which is why I am so surprised that the Old City of Krakow is so beautiful. Stunningly so. The barbican, the castle, the central square—they are all incredible, transporting us to a different time and place with end- less medieval wonder. It's the antithesis of everything we've seen up to this point. The Poles of Krakow took all of the potential aesthetic value of the city and the suburbs and poured it into the tourist center of the city to a greater extent than anywhere we've ever been.

Cassie and I take an evening stroll through the Old City, around the castle, and into the Jewish Quarter, staring up at the church towers and buildings around us that soar into the overcast gray. We spot a Mexican restaurant and decide, for reasons that don't quite make sense now and probably didn't then, that this is what we'll eat tonight.

We've spent the last week in Budapest, Hungary, eating thick, hearty Hungarian foods like langosz—fried dough with sour cream and cheese—or chicken paprikash, a thick, paprika-based sauce served with boiled chicken. With our Hungarian ancestry, it was natural for us to visit, but we had no idea how much we'd love the city. We meant to spend two days there but ended up spending a week without running out of things to do. We visited the second largest Parliament building in the world, soaked in the thermal Turkish baths for an afternoon, explored the largest Jewish temple in Europe, and wandered around the wildly eclectic and bizarre ruin pubs, sipping hot mulled wine. We even met Cassie's cousins for dinner one night, which turned into a bit of a start-and-stop experience since only one of them spoke English and we don't speak a word of Hungarian, short of the few phrases we learned from our free Budapest map. These include yes (*egen*), no (*nem*), and cheers (*egeszsegere*), for which the map gives the helpful tip of saying the English phrase "I guess she can drive" as quickly as possible— despite the completely disparate spellings, you'll come close enough to pronouncing *egeszegere*. Whenever there was a lull in the conversation, which was often, someone would yell *"Palinka!"* and we would all take another sip of their native liquor that tastes like a cross between fresh plums and rancid turpentine—or maybe rancid plums and fresh turpentine.

We had expected that Hungary would be the first departure from what we knew as normal. Our first foray into Eastern Europe would be our first true excursion from Western life, as we left our comfort zones and truly started exploring other countries and cultures. We were somewhat surprised to find out that everything in Budapest was still so . . . Western. Everything felt disturbingly familiar, and we had no problem navigating the city or ordering meals. Even the food was nothing unusual, since we both grew up with Hungarian cooking, which is why, after a week of the thick cuisine of Budapest, we were ready for something other than the borscht and pierogies of Poland.

Hence, Mexican food in the Old City of Krakow. We expected Poland, like Hungary before it, to be very cheap and incredibly affordable. Combine that with the inexpensive Mexican fare we were used to eating in the States, and we assumed we would be eating for dirt cheap. Yet somehow, we end up dining at what might be the most expensive Mexican restaurant in the world, and one where I'm sure no Mexican has ever dined. The food comes as close to authentic Mexican cuisine as General Tso's chicken comes to authentic Chinese cuisine.

A few hours later, we're back at our hostel, ready to call it a night. Even without the other guests staying awake until three in the morning drinking and screaming despite the 11 p.m. quiet time mandate, I'm not sure we would've slept well anyway. The idea of visiting Auschwitz has a way of turning sleep into a disquieting struggle between you and the back of your eyelids.

In the morning, a quick look out the window reveals the weather has cleared. It isn't exactly sunny, but it's no longer the drab airborne bog of the day before. I sleep a little more on the ninety-minute drive to Auschwitz-Birkenau, dreaming that the warmth of the minibus would somehow follow me around the grounds of the largest Nazi concentration camp. I knew that wasn't going to happen before I even woke up. The temperature is in the low forties, and I have the distinct feeling it never gets warm here. Warmth, compassion, friendship—these are all things that left this godforsaken place far behind. Auschwitz is a wasteland of lives and emotions—a complete desolation of the soul—and you can feel it when you approach the gates. We sign up for a guided tour to explore the historic epicenter of evil—the worst genocide in Western history.

As I walk among the buildings and down the pathways, I wonder if my family ever stood where I stand, walked where I walk, and mourned where I mourn. Before the Final Solution, the systematic extermination of Europe's Jews, the Nazis took pictures of many victims. Many of these pictures hang on the walls of certain buildings, and I scan them looking for a familiar face. But I doubt I would recognize my family even if their photographs hung right in front of me; such is the despair on each face. In my mom's photographs, everyone wears an expression of pride. Here, there is none of that.

Our tour guide leads us quickly through Auschwitz—too quickly—before shepherding us to Birkenau. The tour moves too fast for me, and I am left without time to properly reflect or mourn. The guide adds little to the experience, parroting the signs already placed throughout the concentration camp. The visit feels impersonal, even if the subject matter is very intimate. But even a short stay at such a moving place is very powerful. My grandmother's family was here. Somewhere. I've never believed in anything as silly as an Ouija board, but here the dead find a way to speak to you.

We walk quietly through the buildings that once housed the mothers and fathers and brothers and sisters who were about to die. We stare at the remnants of their lives—the clumps of hair, glasses, and cookware that were seized moments after they passed under the *Arbeit Macht Frei* sign— *Work Will Set You Free*. These families thought they were building a new life, unaware the Nazis were about to rob them of their future. I stare at Elsa Meier's faded black chest behind an enclosed display of abandoned luggage. She wrote her address on the exterior that might once have been a rich, dark green, hoping she could identify her belongings after the chaos of arrival. But there was no *after*. We see Klara Sara Focthmann's crushed brown luggage, labeled *Wien* for Vienna. A name is partially revealed from behind a bag, *bermann*, from Hamburg—a distant relative of mine, perhaps.

We see a pile of thousands of confiscated shoes, the vibrant whites and reds long since gone from the dilapidated leather. Prosthetics, braces, and crutches of those deemed unworthy to live even a few more minutes. Outside, rows of empty barracks stand as tombstones in a barren field. A lone flower on a wooden bed built for eight people underscores the hopelessness of this place. There are no birds or squirrels or rats that I can see. No fauna of any kind. Life abandoned this place long ago.

The solitary cattle car used to transport Jews.

The railroad tracks that were the end of the line.

The demolished cremation ovens.

We see it all, walking along the same double-layered barbed wire fences that my family must have walked along decades earlier. I'd like to think they put up a fight or found some way to resist, holding out longer than other prisoners, but I know that's a completely romanticized fiction. They were brought here to die, and they probably died afraid, their will to survive left in the Lodz ghetto from which they came.

In Rome and Barcelona and Paris, we saw what man could accomplish. We saw what people could do. Here, we see the same thing. We see what people can do. We learn what humanity is capable of. In Western Europe, such a lesson was exhilarating. Here, it is horrifying. It will not be the last time on this trip that we reflect on such emotions—we will feel this way again. It would be nice to dream that no such place like Auschwitz exists anywhere else on earth and that people will never let this happen again. That couldn't be further from the truth.

We catch a bus back to Krakow in the late afternoon and decide we need some kind of meal to cheer us up. Visiting Auschwitz is like watching

Black Hawk Down or *American History X* multiplied by a million. Normally I favor beer, but this feels like an opportune time for a bright pastel girly drink with a straw and a tiki umbrella.

Having learned never to trust Mexican restaurants when not in or at least near Mexico, we search for another restaurant. Perhaps more so than any other ethnic cuisine, Mexican food is bastardized and corrupted all over the world. How someone can screw up Mexican food—or Tex-Mex as it often turns out to be—is beyond me. Last time I checked, the dining out equivalent of Mexican food boils down to some combination of five ingredients—tortillas, rice, cheese, veggies, chicken—cooked in one of three ways—baking, frying, or boiling—leaving a very finite number of permutations from which to pick. And yet Mexican food almost always ends up at the top of travel bloggers' lists of ethnic food gone horribly wrong overseas. Tortillas are replaced with fried dough and salsa is replaced with tartar sauce and chicken is replaced with not-chicken. The result is something entirely inedible and not remotely what was intended.

Instead, we find another restaurant. A Mexican restaurant. But at least it more closely resembles what we want. The dishes all have names familiar to any American—burrito, taco, quesadilla—and they even have giant margaritas served in pitchers. We each order one and discover that the only thing the drink has in common with margaritas is the name. Apparently, in Polish, *margarita* means colorful drink. Our pitchers come out in all different shades of neon pinks and blues. The rim, which at first glance seems to be caked in a good, thick layer of salt, is in fact coated in a bulletproof casing of sugar. When we expect the familiar bite of tequila that is at the heart of any good margarita, we detect instead some flavored vodka, masked with more sugar and some sort of fruit juice. I wonder if this drink alone is enough to give me diabetes. The alcohol isn't enough to make us forget the horrors of the morning—there is hardly enough to give us a slight buzz—but the drink personifies bright and peppy, and the food isn't terrible. We spend the rest of the night exploring Krakow and wondering if the drinks will turn our pee glow-in-the-dark blue.

Our time in Europe is winding down. It seems impossible that it's already been two months since we left the States. Soon we'll be leaving for Africa, a place I suspect will feel far less Western than Eastern Europe, but not before we are forced to live through two of the worst transportation experiences of our entire trip.

Two days after Auschwitz, we catch a morning bus to Prague. The schedule says the journey takes ten hours, but that strikes me as odd since Google Maps says it should take only five hours. When we begin moving, I soon find out why this will be the bus ride from hell, far worse than the overnight buses we will take in Vietnam or Southeast Asia. The bus driver stops every twenty minutes. Half the time he picks up passengers, and half the time he stops for a smoke break. We move agonizingly slowly across this stretch of Eastern Europe, inching from one smoke break to the next. Unlike our ride to Krakow, there is no haze to obscure the scenery, and I see each individual tree and shrub pass like molasses across my window. I might have far more sympathy for the bus driver's addiction if I smoked, but given my instinct to avoid inhaling carcinogens, I feel only a deep and unyielding enmity.

We spend a week in Prague—making a quick overnight trip to Vienna—before catching a flight to Naples and a ferry to Sicily for our final week in Europe. The ferry crossing from Naples to Catania sounded like a great idea when Cassie and I planned this part of the trip. We pictured a beautiful overnight sailing excursion down the Tyrrhenian Sea, culminating in a wondrous passage through the Strait of Messina that separates the tip of Italy's boot from the misshapen rugby ball it is about to defenestrate through the narrow aquatic window of the Strait of Gibraltar. It turns into an unending nightmare. We sail straight into a thunderstorm off the Italian coast. The ship, not designed for comfort, is tossed about like a blow-up raft in a typhoon. The bow climbs into the night sky with each new wave, and then crashes down into the dark sea as one wall of water recedes and another approaches. As if the impact of metal upon seawater doesn't make a loud enough thud, the Italians cheer "Oohooopa!" at the top of their lungs at the apex of each liquid sine wave. I wonder if some of them have reverted to their ancestral polytheism and decided now is a good time to taunt Neptune, the Roman god of the sea. But the chants begin to fade. More and more passengers are retiring to their rooms, where they can throw up in private. Cassie is soon among them, leaving our terribly overpriced and horrifically seasoned meal untouched. I don't last much longer. I don't vomit, but I spend the next few hours quietly lying in bed with my eyes closed. This wasn't the romantic ferry journey we had imagined, but it does give me some time to reflect on our time in Europe.

We showed up on the continent with a handful of contacts in disparate cities, but we treated every day as a chance to meet someone new. If sites make a place special, people make it memorable, and we made friends from all over the world during our time here—the Erins and Joshes and Ellens and Marcs and Redas. We had nothing in common with these people except a geographical coincidence and a favorite hobby—we were in the same place at the same time, and we love to travel. In the hours or days we spent together, we built relationships with our new friends that I know will last a lifetime.

Eventually, we both find some comfort in sleep, and the sea is calm when we wake up. I step outside for some fresh air and catch a glimpse of Mt. Etna as we pass through the Strait of Messina.

Chapter 6

December 14, 2013
1°12'58.1"S 36°48'34.3"E
Nairobi, Kenya

There is a natural expectation that people of a certain generation and a particular nationality—a general time and place, if you will—have a high probability of having seen a basic set of movies. For example, if you grew up in 1940s America, you have almost certainly seen *Gone with the Wind* and *Casablanca*. Is that true for everyone? No, absolutely not. But is it true for a large enough subset of the population that I would put money on a randomly picked person from that generation as having seen that movie? Yes, definitely. Similarly, if you consider the 1990s to be the decade when you went from a prepubescent soprano to an adolescent tenor, you have seen, and I say this with a high degree of certainty, *The Lion King*. It was a defining movie for my generation, a beautifully animated adventure combined with a compelling coming-of-age tale in the middle of the African heartland, and it was one of the first movies where it was completely acceptable for boys to admit they cried.

I was in middle school when it came out in 1994, and everyone I know saw it. Everyone but me. I don't know what I was busy doing during those years—other than playing clarinet and computer games—but unfortunately, it did not involve seeing one of the greatest animated movies of all time.

I still bring this up occasionally when my friends and I talk about movies.

"I've never seen *The Lion King*."

"What? Are you serious?"

A sudden gasp noticeably changes the ambient air pressure as everyone spastically inhales, unable to comprehend the words I just strung together into a sentence. In the brief moment before all is forgiven, I am considered less than human, my emotional growth as a child stunted because I did not see a cartoon lion become friends with a cartoon warthog before defeating his cartoon uncle. To people of my generation growing up in the States, not seeing *The Lion King* is akin to not having a complete soul, and maybe it helps explain why I didn't kiss a girl until my junior year of high school.

It is here, in Nairobi, Kenya, that I finally make amends for the egregious transgression in my cinematic choices, which I feel is incredibly appropriate. It also gives me a great excuse from now on when I have to tell people that I didn't see *The Lion King* until I was in my thirties.

"Yeah, I know, it's weird. But I didn't want to see it until I was in Africa and could fully appreciate the emotional weight of the story's underlying metaphors and powerful symbolism."

My nieces insist on watching it with me before we go on our first safari. From what I can gather, a safari is supposed to be exactly like *The Lion King*, only more animals and less singing.

My nieces, of course, didn't move here on their own, since seven- and nine-year-olds rarely switch continents without the express permission and accompaniment of their parents. My older sister, Tamar, moved here in July with her husband, Cam, and their daughters. Cam works for IBM, and they relocated him to Nairobi to manage the company's projects in Africa and the Middle East. He spends most of his time on the road, often visiting places like Lagos, Nigeria, and Dubai in the United Arab Emirates.

They live in Runda Park, an expat community on the outskirts of the dense city center. It is a Western bubble in an African country. Inside my sister's house, it's impossible to tell the difference between Kenya and America. This offshoot of the Liebermann family tree has every modern amenity here. Flat-screen TVs and high-speed Internet. A maid and a gardener. A car and a driver. But the similarities end there. Outside their house, security guards keep watch around the clock. The overnight watchman brings a guard dog. An electrified fence surrounds the property, and the house has its own security system.

My sister's precautions are in no way paranoid or excessive. Every house in the community has its own electrified fence and security guards. The entire compound has an additional electrified fence and another team of security guards at each entrance. All of these guards come from one or two private companies. My sister tells us the cops won't respond unless you offer them a bribe, so you have to make your own private security arrangements.

Karibu Kenya. Welcome to Kenya.

Traffic laws exist only so drivers can ignore them. The local buses, called *matatus*, resemble VW vans, yet fit as many people as London double-deckers. Rumor has it the drivers bribe cops so they have free rein on the roads. Our friends were held up at gunpoint and forced to hand over all of their money and valuables. Foreigners are pulled over and ticketed for violating mystery laws. The tickets "go away" for a sum of Kenyan shillings that the police officer finds acceptable.

This is Africa.

This is Africa. A simple phrase, often uttered with a shrug, that is supposed to both explain the continent's problems and alleviate the tension of whoever is experiencing those problems. From broken-down buses to tribal wars, power outages to genocide, blood diamonds to famine. Why does all this happen here? This is Africa. It is almost a warning to foreigners. Keep your expectations in check. Forethought and planning be damned. Every time I hear someone utter these three words, I get the distinct feeling the continent has given up on itself.

We are the first family members to visit Tamar, and she starts crying when she sees me at the airport. She has close friends here in a tight-knit expat community, but there's nothing quite like seeing family. We tell her all about the trip, showing her pictures of the different cities and countries we visited in Europe, while she tells us all about life in Nairobi. She has no job here but has become incredibly active with her daughters' classes and after-school activities. We take Rachel and Kaila to school every day, and I help Tamar prepare dinner every night for the family. Since the girls have two banana trees in the backyard, I teach them to make banana bread, which becomes a staple in the house.

At some point during my time in Africa, the single most significant event of our entire trip happens. Neither Cassie nor I have any idea that something has irreversibly changed, but my body picks up a virus somewhere. I won't show any symptoms for a few more days, but a medical time bomb has started its relentless countdown, slowly at first, picking up speed in the coming weeks. It will lead me into the hardest days of our trip and the darkest hours of my life. But I don't know it at the time. Instead, Cassie and I settle into our surroundings on a new continent for a few days before it's time for our very first safari.

The rain wakes us up long before my niece knocks on our door. The exact sort of downpour we're hoping to avoid, and here it is, pounding away at Nairobi in biblical proportions. It is the "short rains" season in Kenya, but what the precipitation lacks in duration, it makes up for in unabated intensity. If this doesn't let up, we'll have better luck reaching the plains of the Maasai Mara in an ark. In this part of the world, it would be exceedingly easy to populate the floating wooden domicile with two of each animal. Wildlife thrives here, especially if it hasn't been killed yet for its ivory—a chemical compound no different from human fingernails, which, for reasons that don't make sense to my Western mind, fetches about $1,500 a pound on the black market.

But no, we will stick to our four-row, seven-seat Jeep with not one, but two spare tires. AAA hasn't quite made it to Nairobi yet, let alone the open country outside of Kenya's capital city, so self-sufficiency is of the utmost importance. Nairobi's roads aren't known for drainage or, for that matter, road markings, traffic signs, or any semblance of order. They are, by American standards, complete chaos, but they're the only way for us to get to our destination.

The Maasai Mara is the Kenyan equivalent of Tanzania's somewhat more famous Serengeti. They are essentially the same ecosystem, divided only by an artificial boundary between two neighboring sovereign entities. Kenya has one name for it; Tanzania has another.

We set off on our drive to the Maasai Mara in western Kenya early in the morning—or at least we're about to until a leak renders two-thirds of the rear seats useless. One of the rivets in the roof allows a steady drip of water to seep in and drench the back seat. The subsequent splash soaks the middle seat too. Of course, this is where I'm supposed to be sitting. Evans, our driver and safari guide who looks exactly like Eddie Murphy, pulls a MacGyver and plugs the leak with a toothpick, Mentos chewing gum, and a bit of orange-and-black-patterned duct tape. This is Africa.

For two hours, we drive southwest, away from the crowds of the city and toward the packs of wildlife. Kenya doesn't have speed limits (or at least none that are taken seriously), so they regulate the flow of traffic with speed bumps on even their largest highways. Instead of building pedestrian overpasses, people cross the streets right behind a speed bump, so drivers are at least going marginally slower in the likely event of a collision. Since, if I remember my high school physics class correctly, force equals mass times acceleration, reducing the acceleration appreciably reduces the force, which, in this case, would be taken from a solid metal vehicle and applied to a malleable human body. The human bodies are thankful for this, even if they don't express it as often as they should. Some speed bumps are short and high, others are wide and low. Our driver hurdles these at a variety of speeds that shows no concern for the suspension of the jeep and no correlation to the size of the bumps.

We turn off onto what Evans calls "an African highway," leaving behind the last bit of pavement we will see until the end of our safari. I can't tell if he's being humorous or sarcastic or both, since "African highway" apparently means crater-filled dirt road. Judging by the condition of the road, the asteroid that wiped out the dinosaurs may very well have hit somewhere along this stretch of dirt. The road into the Maasai Mara—which means "spotted plains" in the Maasai language, Maa—is considered one of the worst in Africa, which, one might assume, makes it one of the worst in the world. Evans slows down every few minutes to circumnavigate another ditch or patch of mud or overturned tractor-trailer. His expression remains unchanged. Nothing here surprises him. For us, this is a foreign world. For Evans, this is home.

Along the way, we see poverty as we have never seen it before. Even the poorest person in the poorest county in the poorest state in America wouldn't trade places with the children we see in towns like Seyabei and Ntulele. Clean water is a luxury. Plumbing is a dream. Medicine relies more on ancient herbal remedies than modern scientific research. In one town, the hospital is connected to the butchery, which gives me unpleasant thoughts about both the surgeon's success rate and the butcher's filet du jour. This truly is Charles Dickens's best-of-times-worst-of-times juxtaposition. Living in Runda Park or one of the expat communities near Nairobi is residing in luxury. Living anywhere else in the country is a daily battle with poverty.

My nieces miss the life lesson entirely, burying their attention in their iPads. The next day, mid-safari, one of them will decide seeing two cheetahs eating a zebra is boring, while I think it's one of the most badass things I have ever seen (yes, *badass* is exactly the word to describe it). Instead, my niece watches *Madagascar 2*, passing up the real wild for the animated facsimile. Don't get me wrong. I love animated movies, notwithstanding my failure to see one of the most famous movies of my youth, but this doesn't feel like the time or place to watch one.

The towns, though incredibly poor, are also wonderfully colorful, and I suspect the people living in these towns are far happier than we could ever imagine ourselves to be if we found ourselves in similar conditions. The homes are bright reds and blues and yellows, made even more striking by the gorgeous countryside in the background. Upon closer examination, each home is made of a metal shipping container, which forms the largest component of the makeshift structure, with additional sheets of metal propped up to expand the living area. Some homeowners have repainted their containers Coca-Cola red or Pepsi blue, complete with each soda's ubiquitous logo. The irony is that these families can't even afford the products for which they offer free advertising.

Google says the drive will take four hours and five minutes. Apparently, Google has yet to visit this part of the world. After six hours on the road, we reach the entrance to the Maasai Mara. The rangers greet us in Swahili with a friendly *"Jambo!"* and an *"Asante sana"* after we pay our entrance fees.

A few years ago when Cassie was studying abroad in Mexico, her class visited a local zoo. Inside this zoo was something you would never see back home: an exhibit dedicated to squirrels. Growing up in the United States, this seems absolutely comical, but that's purely a function of how many squirrels we have. There are few, if any, in Mexico, so the squirrels they do have become a tourist attraction. Any American visiting the zoo would laugh at both the squirrels and the people staring at the squirrels.

I suspect that's exactly how Evans feels watching us take hundreds of pictures of zebras. Though certainly more impressive in size and stature, zebras are the African equivalent of squirrels. There are lots of them, and they're not particularly special. They are also, unfortunately for them, at the absolute bottom of the food chain. As Evans tells us all sorts of fun facts about zebras—such as zebra stripe patterns being comparable to finger-prints that uniquely identify each one—Cassie asks, "How long do zebras live?"

Evans doesn't hesitate. "Until the lion finds him." Zebras hold dominion over no one. They are Animalia Soylent Green, eating grass until they are eventually recycled as fertilizer for the grass that will feed more zebras.

Within minutes of entering the Maasai Mara, we spot a black rhino in the distance. Rhinos are solitary and shy, avoiding any real interaction unless you give them a reason to charge. They avoid humans just like they avoid everything else, although our race's propensity for slaughtering them for their horns probably hasn't improved relations between the two species. Our rhino stands alone in a large field, slowly grazing on the grass at his feet at his own pace, oblivious to anything farther away than three feet. I say "our rhino" because no one else is around us to disrupt the moment, and we are left alone to stare at our mammalian friend enjoying his herbivorous lunch.

We have found our first of Africa's Big Five: rhino, lion, elephant, water buffalo, and leopard. These five animals are supposed to consti-tute the pinnacle of safari excitement. Seeing any one of these is cause for popping open some expensive bubbly and laughing merrily at your good fortune. Instead, we simply snap a few pictures with our telephoto lenses, even though they don't have a long enough zoom to get a really good photo of the rhino. Evans says the rhino is male. He proves to us over and over again how good his vision is, spotting animals with his eyes before we see them with binoculars.

Over the next two days, we see three more of the Big Five, as well as countless other animals that didn't make the final cut, like cheetahs, mon-gooses (mongeese?), and giraffes. The leopard, however, eludes us. "You only see a leopard if the leopard wants to be seen," Evans explains as we stare up into yet another tree, hoping to glimpse a hanging tail or animal carcass that would indicate the presence of our evasive friend. We never do, but that doesn't stop us from basking in the breathtaking glory of the Maasai Mara.

We crisscross the wide-open plains in search of animals, and we see wildlife as we have never seen it before. There is no cage here, no veterinarians or staff to care for these animals. They are free here, coexisting in a beautiful balance of teeming life.

On the second day of our safari, we see a pride of lions fighting with a pack of hyenas over a zebra, or rather what's left of a zebra, which consists of most of its head and one hind leg. The lions killed the zebra and are trying to figure out how much more of it they want to eat before allowing the hyenas to take over. The hyenas, which resemble the three, shall we say, "unintelligent" hyenas in *The Lion King* to an extent I would have thought impossible, run around in circles, occasionally trying to snatch a dismembered segment of the zebra. They really do laugh while they're running around in geometrically nonsensical patterns, though it's more of a mad cackle as they are being chased by lions, so the emotional gist of their elocution is probably something other than mirth. A jackal, smaller and far cuter than the other animals, tries to make off with a scrap of the meal. It is a game between the carnivores, and we have a front row seat. I ask Evans if he wants the binoculars. He politely turns me down. He is happy because we are happy. He is showing us the beauty of his homeland. The beauty of Africa.

Occasionally, we have trouble finding something other than zebras and waterbuck. Evans flags down a passing tour group, and the guides chat in Swahili for a few minutes. I'm never quite sure if they're discussing the location of wildlife or the Kenyan soccer team's inability to qualify for the World Cup. Then Evans smiles at us, crosses his fingers, and starts driving. Sometimes we find nothing. Sometimes we find exactly what we're looking for.

I don't take a picture—I take hundreds of pictures. I don't snap a photo of a cheetah—I snap thirty. Later, as I'm looking through pictures from the safari, I find myself asking, "Did I really see this?" I never knew how much a baby elephant clings to its mother. Or how bloodshot a cheetah's eyes look after a kill. Or how tiny a dwarf mongoose really is. You cannot know these things from textbooks or educational videos. You must see them in person to truly understand.

We see the beauty of the Maasai Mara at sunrise and sunset. We see the rains that bring the land to life, hydrating the soil and renewing the earth. We see the Kenya-Tanzania border, and the wide open plains of the Serengeti stretching to the horizon and beyond. We have lunch under a lone tree, surrounded by zebras and waterbuck and giraffes, far away from any sign of other people. We eat our prepackaged meal in the silence of the spotted plains. Sitting here at the edge of the Maasai Mara, farther from home than I have ever been and completely at peace with the world around me, I can't help saying to myself, "This is Africa."

This is Africa.

Chapter 7

December 25, 2013
31°42'15.5"N 35°12'21.6"E
Bethlehem, West Bank

I expected Christmas to be more . . . Christmas-y, especially here in Bethlehem. I didn't think there would be snow or anything like that—this is the Middle East, after all—but I certainly thought there would be a much greater atmosphere of celebration and joy. But standing here in Manger Square, a few feet from the Church of the Nativity where Jesus was born (I would say a stone's throw away, but here in the occupied West Bank, that statement has very different and far more serious implications), I am struck by one thing above all others: how many kids are selling bubble gum.

There are hundreds of them, scampering around Manger Square, greeting tourists briefly before launching into a well-rehearsed sales pitch about the minty flavor of the gum, the delightfully affordable price of a pack, and their need to sell it to maintain an adequate standard of living. I'm not sure if they practice together or if they all learned from the same teacher, because every spiel is nearly identical, from verbiage to intonation.

"Hello! Welcome to Bethlehem. Happy Christmas. Would you like some gum? One shekel. Only one shekel!"

They're offering a really good deal. One shekel for a pack of Doublemint gum works out to about twenty-five cents for five sticks of delectable chewiness. If I have an obligation to accept a good deal, it's certainly here in the Holy Land. You can't get that price anywhere back home. The offer is so good that my Middle Eastern instinct to haggle doesn't kick in immediately. If I invest in their bargain bubble gum, I could make a killing on Doublemint back in the States. I may have hated my finance classes in college, but I certainly understand the concept of buy low, sell high. The only problem is I didn't come here to buy gum. I came here for Christmas.

Cassie and I decided a long time ago that it would be really cool to celebrate Christmas where Christianity began. Forget the fact that I don't celebrate the holiday. That's almost completely irrelevant. You don't need to believe in something to sense the spirituality around it. That's why I'm here, to see some of the most devout Christians in the world making a pilgrimage to Manger Square for the holiday. But the ratio of pilgrims to boys selling bubble gum isn't quite what I expected. This is supposed to be a significant religious event, not a makeshift flea market. Half of the five hundred or so people here are trying to pray, focusing on the liturgy. The other half are doing everything in their power to sell bubble gum to the first half. And so there is a constant drone of prayer, competing with the annoying rattle of sales and marketing. This is, using one of those terrible puns I strive so hard to avoid, a bizarre bazaar.

We spent the day walking around the Old City of Jerusalem, seeing an international menagerie of Christmas traditions on display. Some felt oddly familiar. Holiday lights in Bethlehem look much like holiday lights in the States, and they make us feel as if we're not nearly as far from home as we truly are, separated by both time and distance. Earlier in the day, we caught a Syrian Orthodox parade marching down the narrow, cobbled streets of the ancient city, playing what I can only assume are traditional Syrian Orthodox songs, though how these songs came to be played on Scottish bagpipes I can't possibly fathom, since it requires an intermingling of cultures that I'm quite sure hasn't happened yet.

Here in Jerusalem, we even experienced a bit of a white Christmas. A meter of snow paralyzed the city a few days before the holiday, shutting down the streets and public tram system, and though it melted quickly as temperatures returned to normal, the final remnants of the historic snowfall lingered in the most sun-deprived shadows of the city. Of course, that doesn't compare to the weather back on the eastern seaboard, which is just at the beginning of what will become one of the worst winters on record. We picked a good winter to be very, very far away from home.

We pulled into Bethlehem a few hours ago, sometime in the late afternoon. Technically, I'm not allowed to be here. As an Israeli citizen, it is illegal for me to enter the city, so I carry my American passport in case the border security guards ask. They never do. Bethlehem is a city where it seems anything goes, as long as your ultimate goal is to make a dollar. Or a shekel. The city isn't big enough or commercial enough to draw major corporate investors, so instead of Starbucks Coffee you have Stars and Bucks Cafe. The familiar green female logo has been replaced by a few cups of coffee and swirling steam, all drawn in the same shade of green.

A festive mood permeates the city, and everyone here is celebrating. The narrow streets are packed with honking cars, and there are even a few Santa Clauses whooping and hollering to the crowds. That all changes when we enter Manger Square. It's much quieter here, more somber, and smaller than I expected. My impressions of Christmas revolve heavily around my memory of Rockefeller Center. Big tree, lots of lights, a good deal of singing, maybe even an ice rink. Manger Square lacks most of this, especially the ice rink. There is certainly a big tree, but the heavily armed security guards flanking the evergreen—which may or may not consist of far more artificial plastic than natural pine—somehow detract from the festive mood.

The crowd of pilgrims waits for Midnight Mass, passing the time with Christmas carols from all over the world. Since the group is so diverse and their languages so varied, no more than a few people know each song, and these people inevitably stand in a tight circle with their fellow countrymen, so it sounds like the celebration moves around the square in small pockets of happiness. Fifteen Germans sing *"Weihnachtslieder"* at the northeast corner of the square, followed by ten Finns singing *"Joulun kellot"* off to my left, and then thirty Ukrainians chime in with *"Boh predvichnyi narodyvsia"* somewhere to the west.

We find a dinner spot at a tourist restaurant that overlooks the square. The waiter serves up baked chicken in a brown sauce that I'm quite sure would make a distinct slopping sound if dropped from a height of three inches or more. Sometime in the near future, we should be visiting the Church of the Nativity—possibly the oldest church in Christianity—before settling in for a few hours to wait for Midnight Mass. The only problem is that our tour group didn't anticipate the VIPs that would also be visiting the Church of the Nativity to pay their respects on this evening, which means the church is closed to anyone who's not Fouad Twal, the Latin Patriarch of Jerusalem, or a ranking member of a government or embassy. That leaves us to while away the time eating dinner and walking around the streets of Bethlehem, with the unfortunate consequence that we run out of stuff to do fairly quickly. Apparently, there's only so much fun one can have haggling down the price of a pack of gum.

As much as we'd love to stick around for the penultimate Catholic service, we decide to hop on the early bus leaving town at 10 p.m., especially since we'd have to watch the service in a language we don't understand on a screen we can't quite see in a city I shouldn't be in. Latin class couldn't keep me awake in high school, which makes it highly unlikely that I'll understand any of what's being said now, never mind the fact that my religion doesn't subscribe to the story that the Almighty has or had any offspring to which we should be offering prayers on a holiday that celebrates his birth while missing the actual date by at least two full seasons. Getting a good night's rest seems the prudent option.

We spend the next few days driving in circles between Jerusalem, Tel Aviv, and Haifa, visiting my cousins and catching up with everyone. We have no intention of seeing the group of cousins who won't see us, which works out in a wonderful mutually exclusive sort of way where we can ignore each other in peace. After New Year's Eve, we make our way down to Eilat, the southernmost point in Israel, for some snorkeling and an overnight trip to Petra, the ancient kingdom in the Jordanian desert. The five-hour drive takes us through the Negev Desert into some of the most inhospitable terrain in Israel. Much of this land is so barren it makes for an excellent bombing range, and it's not uncommon to see Israeli Air Force jets streaking by at low altitude after dropping practice munitions. On the way down, I gorge on a box of six Krembos.

I cannot adequately describe my love for Krembo, and after my pedestrian description, I'm sure you won't be rushing to find a package. That's a shame, since they're absolutely divine. Imagine a thin cookie, no more than two inches across, with a mound of a substance that's not unlike sweetened whipped cream, but it holds together at room temperature. Now dip that whole thing in a very thin layer of chocolate. There, you have a

Krembo. It comes in vanilla and mocha flavors, and each one is heavenly for its own reasons. Instead of soda or sunflower seeds to keep me awake during the drive, I eat a Krembo every hour or so, waiting until the joy of one has faded and I can no longer resist the urge to eat another one.

Before long, we exit the nothingness that is the desert and enter the gleaming city of Eilat. When my parents honeymooned here a few decades ago, Eilat was the sort of quiet getaway town that people might enjoy. Now, it's full of glamorous hotels and shopping plazas that make it everything we want to avoid on our world trip. But I still have very fond memories here from previous trips to Israel, and that makes it too much to pass up. Eilat is also one of the best spots from which to visit Petra.

On a free day in the city, we head for a reef and rent snorkels. The water is so salty—far more so than the ocean but not nearly as salty as the Dead Sea—that we float effortlessly, bobbing our way from one submerged chunk of reef to the next. The reefs are divided between adjacent beach clubs, and you access the water via a long walkway that extends over it and ends in three steps leading you into the Red Sea. We hop into the water at one end of the beach clubs, float with the current to the other end, and walk out along another gangway. It's delightfully easy, and we make the trip a few times, picking different spots over which to float. The water is a bit choppy, and every once in a while a slightly larger wave submerges the end of my snorkel, gagging me with a mouthful of water that contains enough sodium chloride to be very unpleasant. In a few trips along the reef, I drink more than my fair share of the Red Sea.

Even if Eilat isn't considered one of the world's greatest reefs, it's still majestic. On one trip down the reef, I find myself surrounded by a school of fish, completely oblivious to me or to the destruction I could do to their population if I had a fishing rod and some bait. Another school of fish engulfs me on the next dip, until I realize it's probably the same school of fish being exactly as oblivious to me as they were just a few minutes ago. Still, it's very exciting the second time around, and I hope that, with their short memory, it's just as exciting for them.

The air is far colder than the water, so the decision to repeat the same floating snorkeling excursion is more a consequence of our desire to stay warm than of being infatuated with the underwater life. Alas, after three trips along the same patch of reef, we decide it's time to retreat to the warmth of the showers and the changing room.

"You look like you've lost some weight," Cassie says to me casually as we make our way back to our rental car.

"Great! I've been meaning to drop a few pounds." I think nothing more of the conversation, and I barely waste any time trying to figure out how I ate thousands of calories of delicious, chocolate-dipped sugar yesterday, yet find myself shedding pounds today.

The following morning finds us on a bus to Petra. Or, more accurately, on a bus to the Israel-Jordan border and the southernmost border crossing. It takes two hours to hand over our passports, wait for the stamps, retrieve our passports, hand them to someone else wearing a different flag on his shoulder, wait for the stamps, and again retrieve our passports before we're allowed to hop on an entirely different bus for the drive into Jordan.

If Rockefeller Center determined my predispositions about Christmas festivities, then *Indiana Jones and the Last Crusade* colored my thinking about Petra. A long, narrow valley in the shape of a crescent moon suddenly opens up into the lost city of Petra, its buildings carved out of the valley's rose-colored rocks. Inside, we can expect to find a similarly lost seven-hundred-year-old knight guarding a dazzling collection of wine cups, one of which may be the Holy Grail. Drinking from the wrong chalice will find us shriveling away as our hair grows very long and wiry in only a few seconds' time. Drinking from the right chalice will grant us eternal life. I hope my expectations aren't too high.

Petra isn't the only lost city in this region. The Middle East has a nasty habit of misplacing its cities. In some cases, these cities are rediscovered after a few millennia. Sometimes, they remain lost. Take Masada for example. The ancient city by the Dead Sea claimed a group of Byzantine monks as its last inhabitants around the fifth or sixth century. It went missing for the next 1,300 years until it was found in 1838, give or take a few years. Archaeologists rejoiced, and UNESCO added it to the list of world heritage sites in 2001, joining Petra, which was added in 1985. Meanwhile, Ur, the biblical city of Abraham, was abandoned in 500 BC when the Babylonian empire fell to the Persian empire, just as the Iron Age was really hitting its stride. It was AWOL for more than two millennia. By the time Ur was discovered and identified in 1853 in modern-day Iraq, the Industrial Revolution was winding down.

Petra follows this historic if somewhat regrettable tradition of misplacing urban centers. The city was abandoned in 663 AD, forgotten for the next 1,200 years, and rediscovered by Europeans in 1812. Based on this track record, I half expect Atlantis to be waiting for an amateur archeologist armed with a Dora the Explorer backpack to flip over a rock or turn a corner and discover the city somewhere in the Middle East after a few hundred more years have passed.

Our bus driver drops us off at the gift shop that marks the beginning of the trail down to Petra. Gift shops are the universal indicators that something interesting is nearby. Any place of historic value—and quite a few places that have absolutely no value—are marked by a gift shop. The relative importance of the location can be judged by the number of shops, the collection of knick-knacks they sell, and how far away they are from the point of interest. The Great Wall of China, for example, has large clusters of well-stocked gift shops that radiate out quite far from the Wall itself. The Mitchelstown Caves in Ireland, on the other hand, have only one gift shop at the ticket counter that sells the smallest possible collection of postcards.

The first small tent we see sells a bewildering array of postcards, hookahs, and random assorted junk that can only be described as tchotchkes. It is cleverly called INDIEANA JONES GIFT SHOP. They definitely know how to cash in on marketing here, even if the promotions strategy is a bit outdated. We line up with our tour group and follow the signs to the once-lost-but-now-found city. The path to Petra descends through beautiful swirling red rock formations that seem otherworldly in a truly entrancing way. The rock walls of the gorge look like they've been shaped and polished by a master of modern art, whirling and dipping with a chaotic sense of beauty. As we make our way toward the ancient city, we begin to see a hint of the buildings ahead. Ancient rock carvings that have miraculously stood up to the withering forces of centuries of wind and sand adorn some of the rock walls, peeking out as if this ghost city is ready to come to life once again.

The final steps through a narrow fissure and into the fabled city are exactly as awesome and dramatic as Indiana Jones makes it seem. The famous rock facade of Petra becomes gradually visible as you inch closer to the site, its full majesty hidden until the very last moment. Its size is breathtaking.

Cassie and I spend more than a few minutes staring at the facade, known as the Treasury, even though it almost certainly wasn't a treasury.

Petra is a wonder of ancient engineering and art, and I think the Nabataeans who claimed the city as their capital had a healthy amount of common sense, some of which I'm sure we could use today. Instead of doing what other city-builders did for thousands of years and moving the rock to the city, the Nabataeans (or at least their architects) realized it would be far easier to move the city to the rock. They didn't have to carve out stones to build a castle. They simply took the stone that was already formed all around them and carved the city straight into the rock, and they did it in an incredible fashion, with intricately detailed decorations far above ground level. The Nabataeans also built a system of cisterns and floodgates to control the flash floods that occasionally plague the area. They built an oasis in the middle of the desert that stands to this day.

After three hours exploring this wondrous city, the fun part of this trip comes to an abrupt end. Our tour package was supposed to include a night in a hotel. *Hotel* is a term that conjures up images of warm, neatly made beds and hot showers, possibly even a breakfast buffet with eggs and yogurt. *Hotel* does not in any way describe the isolated tent city where our bus stops. For a brief moment, I get very excited when I realize we may be staying in a Bedouin village. That excitement soon fades into a mild sort of growing displeasure when it becomes readily apparent that this is, instead, a few cheap tents carefully designed to depict a Bedouin village without, in fact, having any real Bedouin.

The Bedouin are a nomadic desert people known for their legendary hospitality. If a traveler comes by a Bedouin encampment, he will be welcomed in without a moment's hesitation and treated to endless amounts of water, food, tea, and anything else the village has to offer.

I experienced this hospitality back in college, when I signed up for a Birthright Israel trip, mostly so I could score a free flight to Israel. One of the most unique experiences was a night we spent in a Bedouin camp. I'll never forget the breakfast they served us. A delectable smorgasbord of fresh pita and yogurt and chocolate milk and eggs and on and on.

It becomes obvious very quickly that this isn't the sort of hospitality we should expect. First, there is no offer of food and water. Our group, consisting of a few Americans, a Norwegian, and three Italians, has to ask for our meal after sitting at the table for a good thirty minutes being completely ignored by the hosts. After a few more minutes, we realize water apparently isn't included in the meal, so we have to ask for that too. Second, the only fire, which is also the only source of heat, is a small bonfire burning in one corner of the main tent area. Four or five Jordanians monopolize the space around the fire and its warmth, leaving us shivering in the frigid evening air of the Wadi Rum desert. They pay far more attention to their hookah pipes than to us.

It's not that I have any problems staying in a tent with Jordanians masquerading as Bedouin nomads. Quite the opposite—a night in the desert sounds pretty exciting and wild, perhaps even a little exotic. My only problem is staying in a tent in the middle of the desert when I expected a hotel.

In the middle of the night, I find myself having to go to the bathroom. Of course, there is no bathroom in my tent, so I have to walk a few minutes from our semi-private enclosure to the camp's main area. As soon as I leave the relative warmth of my tent and step outside, I instantly regret my decision. No need to use the latrine is great enough to justify dealing with these freezing temperatures, but having come this far already—all the way to the other side of our tent flap—I might as well finish the journey to the water closet and back.

The bathroom, designed to accommodate the crowds that presumably arrive in tourist season, is a stark reminder that we are in a biblical land. I say that because it appears the flood waters in the time of Noah's Ark have just now begun to recede in the bathroom. Everything is wet, far too wet to explain with something as simple as "a faucet exploded" or "someone has been showering for three whole days." Nothing short of forty days and forty nights of constant rain could possibly explain how much water there is in this bathroom, maybe even enough to turn this entire desert into arable land. I relieve myself, shuffle back to bed while skirting around Pacific Ocean-esque formations of water on the floor, and await the coming dawn.

I already knew not to expect a true Bedouin breakfast at this tentpocalypse. But in all of my notes from the trip and all of the other moments and memories I have pieced together from Petra, I cannot for the life of me remember what they served us for breakfast. I suspect this is because of what happened immediately after breakfast when it was time to head back to Israel. Before we leave, which is to say, before we are allowed to leave, we are kindly informed that we have to pay for the water we drank with dinner last night.

"One dinar each water," our hosts tells us. For us, this is a not insignificant problem. We normally carry around at least a bit of the local currency. In Israel, we always had shekels; in Prague, korunas; in Poland, zlotys. But we were told we wouldn't need any money on this tour unless we wanted to buy some souvenirs, so we never exchanged dollars for dinars. The one time we did buy something—a blue and white scarf at a gift shop—we paid with a credit card, which wasn't a problem at all since we were willing to pay an extra dinar for the cost of using plastic. Never in my wildest dreams did I think our hosts would charge us for water, especially when they offered us nothing else to drink with dinner. When we explain this dilemma to our host, he offers his own version of a solution.

"One of you pay me now. Everyone else pay him later," he says, shrugging. I knew the desert was a harsh environment. I just didn't know how harsh. Our host doesn't care who knows who or how we're all connected or if we'll ever see each other again. He just wants to get paid. Thankfully, the Norweigan in our group has the dinars to cover the waters, and we pay him back in shekels once we return to Eilat.

The rest of our time in Israel winds down quickly. We have only a few days before we move east once again. We have completed the Europe, Africa, and Middle East portions of our trip. Now we head for the Far East and Nepal. Western civilization is in our rearview mirror. According to our plans, we will not see a familiar face again for five months.

Chapter 8

January 9, 2014
13°44'07.6"N 100°30'42.8"E
Bangkok, Thailand

In some parts of the world, getting lost is an acceptable, perhaps even a desirable, thing to do. We thoroughly enjoyed wandering around Venice's myriad alleys and canals without any clue as to where we were or where we were going. We spent a wonderful afternoon meandering through the labyrinthine streets of Paris, breathing in the cafe culture of one of Europe's best cities. But never in a million years would I recommend getting lost in Bangkok. And not just a bit lost. I mean, I have no f'ing idea where we are. We are somewhere in the middle of one of the largest cities in Southeast Asia, a metropolis of fifteen million people.

In Western imaginations, Bangkok is known primarily for two things: incredible street food and a booming sex industry. For the equivalent of ten American dollars, you can buy a plate of panang curry and see a young lady . . . well, never mind.

I have decided not to finish the previous sentence. Well, that's not totally true. I did finish it. Then I read it once or twice and promptly deleted every word that came after it. If this book is ever made into a movie, the second half of that sentence alone will make the movie inappropriate for most audiences. More importantly, if that's the sort of literature you're looking for, then you almost certainly aren't going to want to read this book.

On our first night in Bangkok, we venture out in search of pad thai and spicy noodle soup. Every one of our friends who has been to Bangkok—a list far shorter than I just made it sound—had raved about how delicious and cheap the street food was, and we were determined to find out for ourselves if they were exaggerating.

We ask the girl at the front desk of our hostel where to find good street food, and she points us toward Chinatown. We figure she has to know what she's talking about, because there are all sorts of street food stalls lined up outside of our hostel, but she doesn't direct us to any of those.

During the twenty-minute walk to Chinatown, Bangkok blows away every single one of our assumptions about Southeast Asia. We expected a small city, maybe some one-story buildings, and neighborhoods that resembled shantytowns more than urban dwellings. We basically expected Bangkok to resemble Nairobi, but with better food.

We couldn't have been more wrong.

Bangkok is an ultra-modern city with its own collection of skyscrapers, congested streets, and angry cab drivers. No urban environ can claim to be a real city unless it has its own assortment of angry cab drivers, which is why Philadelphia, Pennsylvania, is a very real city while Rhodes, Greece—which was named the city with the friendliest cab drivers according to a British survey—is not.

We wander down streets with names that make absolutely no sense to us—names like Thanon Charoen Krung and Phra Phiphit—hoping that we find something that identifies these streets as Chinatown, then hoping that we find something on these streets that resembles a street food cart. Unfortunately, neither of those things seems particularly likely to happen at this moment for a multitude of reasons, not the least of which is that we don't speak Thai.

I have absolutely no idea where we are. We should be in the general vicinity of Chinatown, but "general vicinity" means one thing in Duluth, Minnesota, and entirely another in Bangkok, Thailand. I wouldn't worry about the former. I currently find myself quite concerned about the latter.

As a general rule, one of the most important things to do when you're completely lost in a foreign city is to make sure you don't look like you're completely lost in a foreign city. But it becomes appallingly obvious that we're doing exactly that at this moment. We wander in circles around the same few streets, trying to find anything that says Chinatown or anyone who looks like they may consider selling us a plate full of noodles they whipped up on the curb. We strike out on both of those objectives repeatedly. We find ourselves hungry and lost in a foreign city, 8,653 miles from home.

A nice old lady walks up to us out of nowhere and asks us in very good English if we're lost. We kindly reply that we are, and that we're looking for street food.

She tells us to follow her. She will take us to a good street food place. We ask her, "Are you sure?"

"Yes, I'll take you. I'm on my way to church."

Alarm bells go off in my head. It's fairly late on a random weeknight, and this equally random lady is going to lead us to a street food place out of the generosity of her heart? This sounds too good to be true. As she takes us down dark streets and back alleys, I become convinced that I will end up in a bathtub full of ice with one or both of my kidneys missing. That's how all these stories end. For once, I don't think I'm being overly skeptical about human nature because I spent eight years reporting. I may not be skeptical enough right now. She may not even anesthetize me before surgically removing my kidney(s).

In four months on the road, we have only encountered one scam. A guy in Paris "found" a gold ring on the ground in front of us and tried to convince us to buy it. We didn't bite. Before traveling, we trained ourselves to always be on guard against scams. But here we are, on our first night in Bangkok, and it's starting to look an awful lot like another scam. And we have no idea how this one will end.

Our spontaneous tour of Bangkok's seediest streets continues with no sign of ending, at least not in the friendly, congenial way in which many tours are supposed to end: a woman in a weathered smile and company T-shirt tells us to enjoy our day and kindly points us to the receptacle into which we should place our tips. That's not happening anytime soon. I'm not sure if it's just my imagination or if the streets are really getting darker and narrower. We make a bewildering array of rights and lefts as we hurtle after this woman. If our guide's intention is to get us even more lost than we already are, she has succeeded beyond her wildest expectations. It's at times like this that I understand the genius behind Hansel and Gretel leaving behind a path of breadcrumbs to follow home, even if their shortsightedness in failing to anticipate the birds eating their bread crumbs was, to put it mildly, regrettable. Or Theseus using a ball of string to track his way through the minotaur's maze. They were geniuses of foresight. We are about to pay for our stupidity with our lives.

After about ten minutes of walking down random streets, our host stops and smiles at us. This is it. My final moments of consciousness before I am drugged and parted from my kidneys. I'm not sure if Cassie understands everything that's about to happen. She seems very nonchalant about this whole thing, as if she's not nearly as suspicious as I am.

"We're here." Before us is a small establishment, not quite a street food vendor, but not a full restaurant either. The cook prepares the food in a large cart positioned on the sidewalk, then serves it to the patrons seated at a few indoor tables. I am beyond relieved that we have arrived at a legitimate restaurant, especially when I notice the conspicuous absence of surgical equipment. This kind, random lady really did lead us to street food after all.

No one at this restaurant speaks English, so the lady takes us inside, grabs us a seat, and starts making food recommendations. At this point, I become convinced she's going to ask us to buy her food. I wouldn't mind, because I know from months of travel that no foreign help is free. Everyone wants to be paid, especially when the currency is American dollars.

She points at food others have ordered and describes what's in it and how spicy it is. She doesn't think much of our Western ability to handle Thai spices, so she orders our meals for us, making sure we sample a variety of tastes and plates. She tells us that the table next to us is a group of her fellow church members. After we order, she makes sure our waiter doesn't try to rip us off on the check. The food is absolutely fantastic, and she chats amiably with us while we masticate our way through the different dishes.

A series of somewhat related but completely random thoughts run through my mind. Primarily, what the heck is happening? Secondarily, who is this lady and why haven't we cloned her yet? Tertiarily, is everyone in Thailand this nice? We have trained ourselves to believe that stuff like this simply doesn't happen to Western backpackers. You are always the target of a scam and everyone is always out to get you, maybe not in a violent way, but because they love your currency, whether it's dollars or euros or pounds. Those assumptions seemed to work well up until this very evening, when they all fall apart in a blaze of Thai friendliness—and not the kind that involves ladyboys and Ping-Pong balls.

A few minutes later, the woman excuses herself and is about to leave when we ask her for a quick picture. Not once does she ask for food, money, or our kidneys. She is being good to us because she wants to. She is a genuinely kind person.

As we talk about the evening back in our hostel, we realize we don't know the woman's name. She will always be a stranger to us, and yet we will always consider her our friend. How is that possible? I have no idea. It doesn't make sense—and it makes perfect sense. It shouldn't have happened. But it happened.

It's not all that uncommon to find a stranger willing to help in a foreign country—though not as common as finding a stranger ready to rip you off—but this woman didn't just help us for a few moments. She completely devoted herself to our cause for an hour or more, even if that cause was simply finding a decent bite to eat for two famished travelers. In my book—the figurative book in my mind, not this actual book—that is perhaps the most noble of causes.

I'm still not aware of what's happening inside my body, and I dismiss the constant thirst as a consequence of the relentless heat of Bangkok. I've never experienced heat like this before, and I am always drinking water or buying a fresh coconut for a dollar or a fruit shake for two dollars to quench my thirst. My body is breaking down, still slowly, but that's about to change. I will unknowingly accelerate the deterioration of my entire system with one of the most exciting parts of our entire year. As we race around the globe, I am racing toward my own personal judgment day faster than I can imagine.

We spend three more days wandering around Bangkok, exploring the Golden Palace and the world's largest reclining Buddha while eating as much street food as possible. We never visit Patpong, which is Bangkok's internationally famous red light district. It's not that we have no interest in seeing that area—as a journalist, I am obligated to be interested, or at least that's the excuse I was ready to use in case someone snapped any compromising pictures of me—but we simply run out of time in a city that offers so much to see and do and eat. It's a shame that we don't have more time to explore Bangkok, but we will be back in a few weeks to explore the rest of Thailand when we begin our Southeast Asia tour. For now, our next stop is Nepal.

Chapter 9

January 17, 2014
28°31'43.5"N 83°53'44.3"E
En Route to Annapurna Base Camp,
  Western Region, Nepal

I never expected that hiking in the Himalayas would be easy. Even the phrase "hiking in the Himalayas" presents an alliterative difficulty that you can't say five times fast without stumbling. Performing any sort of activity in a location where the altitude requires five digits to the left of the decimal place is incredibly challenging, and I knew that when we signed up for our excursion into the world's most imposing mountain range.

I just never thought it would be this hard.

Each step is impossible. Every inch feels like a marathon. And I have a long way to go until we reach our destination: Annapurna Base Camp. A small cluster of guest houses tucked into the Himalayas, high in the Annapurna range. No power, no heat, and, when the temperature drops below freezing and turns the water in the pipes to ice, no running water. Yet there is something about it that sounds delightfully charming.

Annapurna Base Camp is our stated goal, the reason we've been hiking for four days. Our motivation for waking up early this morning and skipping breakfast is so we can make it to ABC, as it's commonly called, relax for a few minutes, enjoy what we have accomplished, have a quick breakfast, and start our descent.

Maybe it's because I haven't eaten breakfast. My body has become accustomed to tea and porridge with fruit every morning. It's not a massively nutritious serving of edibles, but it's a hiker's meal. Enough food for fuel, but not so much it weighs you down. Now, without the benefit of calories to burn, I'm absolutely gassed. My speed registers one step above crawling, plodding along like a crippled three-toed sloth. Every movement is deliberate. Right foot forward. Left trekking pole forward. Left foot forward. Right trekking pole forward. Repeat.

Maybe it's the altitude. We're up at thirteen thousand feet, higher than I've ever been before. I grew up at the luxury of sea level, and my house was only a fifteen-minute bike ride to the New Jersey beaches, so my lungs are used to a rich, endless supply of oxygen molecules per cubic meter. Four days ago, our hike started at three thousand feet, which wasn't too bad at all. And it wasn't bad for the next two days, until we crossed ten thousand feet. At these elevations, everything becomes harder, gradually at first, and now all at once.

Or maybe it's that I'm out of shape. The simplest explanation is often the right one. Sure, we walked all around Europe, but this isn't Europe. Italy and France and Spain have no mountains compared to the Himalayas, and certainly not where we were in those countries. Towering peaks surround us in every direction, reminding us how difficult and how inhospitable this area has been since the very inception of human history. Eight of the ten highest mountains in the world are within a few hours of us. Annapurna I—the mountain toward which we relentlessly climb—was the first eight-thousand-meter peak ever climbed, three years before Everest. The Alps don't compare. Neither do the Rockies. Nor the Andes. And don't even mention the Adirondacks.

Not once do I imagine that something far worse is happening inside my body.

When I can't move fast enough to warm up my body, my hands start freezing through my gloves. I pound my hands together, put them in my pocket, and pump my arms up and down, but nothing works. My hands are beyond feeling cold. They hurt like hell. Our guide gives me his gloves to put over my own, and the pain of nearly frostbitten fingers slowly subsides. More than once, I think I won't make it. Can't make it. Cassie is well ahead of me, and I am barely lumbering along. When Cassie looks back, she thinks I'm not moving.

I pray in every language I know, and when I run out of prayers, I make up new languages to pray in. We are hiking in fresh snow, and every few steps I punch through a layer of snow and find myself standing in three feet of bone-numbing cold. I had laboriously dried everything the night before, but every stitch of clothing is wet again. The snow soaks my pants, my shoes, and then my socks. This wasn't exactly the hike I had in mind when we signed up to volunteer in Nepal.

We landed in this country five days ago and were immediately assaulted by a small army of Nepali cab drivers at Kathmandu's Tribhuvan International Airport. They wield a mob mentality as their blunt-edged weapon, swarming every foreigner immediately after clearing customs. They insist you put down your backpack, right here, yes please, thank you, only so they can pick it up, carry it five feet, and demand a tip for their service. Whoever picked it up gets the tip. Every other cab driver yells at you, screams at you, and berates you to give him the tip. We are immune to their guilt-tripping shenanigans, but the Chinese college students who share a bus with us succumb to the insanity and hand over a small wad of Nepali rupees.

Nepal made our list of countries from the very beginning because it was our chance to volunteer. Although we've always believed that anyone who wants to travel can make it happen, that really only applies to Westerners and people from developed, relatively wealthy countries. Our minimum wage of $7.25 an hour amounts to a small fortune in most countries. So, in exchange for us being able to see the world, we wanted to give back.

A few years ago, Cassie considered teaching English to Buddhist monks in Nepal for a summer. She found Alliance Nepal, a volunteer organization, and spoke with the manager, Krishna Timilsina, but wasn't able to commit to that much time abroad. While planning our trip, Cassie reconnected with Krishna to arrange our volunteering stay. We signed up to teach for five weeks, then hike for one.

Krishna made all of our transportation arrangements. We spent one night in Kathmandu before hopping on a bus to Pokhara, the town where we would stay. The bus ride is only about 150 miles, but that equates to a full day of travel in Nepal. The eight-hour bus ride lurches along some of the steepest, most twisted roads I've ever seen, barely wide enough for our decrepit vehicle to navigate. When we pull into the Pokhara bus park, Krishna is waiting for us, standing next to his motorbike. After months of exchanging emails, we are thrilled to finally meet. He is a foot shorter than me and half my size, which describes nearly every one of the twenty-seven million people in Nepal. His body language displays the reticence of a culture not used to physical interaction—any American would consider his handshake half-hearted, which is only exacerbated by his rail-thin fingers—and his smile never quite fills his face, but he is warm and welcoming, and his English is excellent. He speaks with a slight Nepali accent, which in most ways resembles an Indian accent.

We follow him in a cab to Lakeside, the tourist district in Pokhara, made up of guest houses and restaurants that all claim to have the fastest Wi-Fi in the city, a mathematical impossibility that seems to bother no one. Even in the nicest section of the city, we are light-years away from Western amenities. Cows wander the streets, leaving steaming piles of excrement in their wake. Considered sacred by Hindis, the cows here are immune from any form of persecution, and they lazily zigzag along the dust-covered roads. Or sit down in the middle of a busy street. Or shit on the street. Or chase each other down a sidewalk. It is the sort of life I may aspire to one day.

If there is a Nepali national anthem, I conclude within a few minutes of arrival that it must be the blast of the car horn. Every driver beeps constantly at other drivers, at people, and at nothing in particular—but never at cows. The sort of reverence we have for luxury cars or fine wines they save for *bos taurus indicus*. One guide book even recommends experiencing and enjoying the car horns as a way of showcasing the personality of a car and its driver. This is patently hogwash. The horns are an endless assault on my eardrums.

Krishna sets us up in one of the guest houses on the main street near Phewa Lake and lays out our next few days. We have two days of sightseeing in Pokhara before we begin trekking.

"I thought we were supposed to do our hike after volunteering?"

"It will be too late. It is winter in the Himalayas, and there will be too much snow. You will hike on Wednesday," he says matter-of-factly. We have been sealed to our fate. We will hike on Wednesday. I've been feeling a little tired lately, but there's no use in trying to switch our hike to the end of our time in Nepal. We don't have the equipment to hike in bad weather.

Between seeing the sun rise over the Himalayas in the nearby village of Sarangkot and taking a short class in Nepali, we grab the last few supplies we need for the eight-day trek and buy a few Snickers bars to celebrate at the end of each day of hiking.

We meet our guide and porter on the way to Naya Pool, a trekker's checkpoint that marks the beginning of the trail to Annapurna Base Camp. There is, of course, a varied menagerie of gift shops. Naya Pool—or Nayapool or Nayapul or Naiapool, depending on who made the sign—is a tourist town. Its sole purpose is to feed trekkers who are just starting or just finishing their hikes.

Laxmi is in his early twenties, an independent trekking guide who has hiked to all of the nearby sites many times. He is confident, both in his trekking skills and in his English. He has led trekkers from all over the world to ABC, and he already has a plan for us, which he cheerfully shares with a bravado that is rare for Nepalis. His international hikers have rubbed off on him. He wears a gray imitation North Face jacket and a backpack that looks like it was made for a few books instead of a few days of trekking.

Tulasi, our porter, is around the same age, and he shoulders the weight of our main pack. He is half my size yet carries twice my weight. Two sleeping bags, two small bags of clothing, our toiletries, and his own bag. I thought the combined weight of our gear might break his back. He proves me wrong very quickly, walking faster than us downhill and nearly as fast uphill.

The first day is hot, the rays of the mid-afternoon sun adding just a little more weight to our packs. We stop often for short water breaks, but we're moving well. Laxmi announces that we will eat lunch at Birethanti, one of many small, nearly identical guest towns along the hike that cater to backpackers. Over the course of the hike, we will gain more than ten thousand feet, and each step up brings us a few inches higher into the Himalayas.

From the very beginning of the hike, the trail is narrow and clogged with donkeys. The donkeys deposit piles of their manure along the trail as they walk, which their hoofs then pulverize into a fine dust that covers the path and the grass on either side. Between the donkeys, we pass supply porters, Nepalis who make a living ferrying supplies up the mountain. Many of them walk barefoot, supporting the weight of food and drinks slung across their back with a strap around their forehead. That seems physically impossible to me, but they do it with the sort of ease that makes me want to visit the gym immediately and repeatedly. One even carries a cage with dozens of chickens on his back, hauling the birds into the mountains for their eggs and their meat. It's humbling to see how effortlessly they pass us, barely breaking stride as they circumnavigate our little group of four inching along the trail.

After two hours of hiking, we see Birethanti and hike the final few minutes to our restaurant. Within twenty feet of the table, my left calf cramps, forcing me to stretch before I grab my seat.

"It's okay, babe. I'll be fine," I tell Cassie, packing all of the confidence I can into my voice.

Every meal we eat always starts with some sort of tea. Black tea, ginger tea, lemon tea, masala tea. Your choice. But always tea. I become somewhat addicted to tea during the hike. Most nights I order a big pot of tea, partly to keep warm and partly because I can't stop drinking it. I pay for my gluttony in the worst way possible, having to go to the bathroom in the middle of the night in the Himalayas. None of our rooms have toilets, so we have to climb out of our sleeping bags, put on some clothing, find our headlamp, and brave the freezing cold nighttime temperatures to go to the bathroom. In my half-awake state, I have to use a Nepali toilet—little more than a glorified hole in the ground—without slipping on the wet porcelain edge of the latrine.

At lunch, I order some vegetable momo, which are little Nepali dumplings, steamed or fried. We eat our meals and rest a bit. Laxmi smiles at me. "Now we begin the steep part," he says, grinning and pointing at the jagged stone stairs that lead away from the restaurant.

The cramps strike immediately, paralyzing first my left leg, then my right leg. My calves, my quads, and all sorts of muscles I didn't know I have lock up. I try to make all sorts of excuses. I'm dehydrated. I'm tired. I'm trying to be a vegetarian in Nepal and don't have enough protein. The true explanation is of course the simplest. I'm out of shape for this sort of trekking. Cassie and I had walked all around Europe, but nothing prepared us for this.

I stop as often as I can, stretching the cramps out of my legs, only for them to come back with a vengeance. When Laxmi declares we are nearing our stop for the night in Ghandruk, I try to move faster, hoping to reach our guest house before I can't walk anymore.

Big mistake. My entire left leg locks, cramping all the way from my hip to my foot. I can barely take a step without falling over. With only a few feet to go, I suddenly can't walk. In sight of our guest house, I have to take another break.

When I'm finally able to relax with a cup of tea at night, I keep thinking the same thing over and over.

This is day one.

To say that we climbed 10,000 feet to Annapurna Base Camp during our hike is both accurate and misleading. We certainly went from 3,000 to 13,500 feet, but we also crossed three valleys, meaning we had to descend one mountain and ascend another mountain. In the end, we climbed much more than 10,000 feet before we encountered the hardest three hours of my life *and* one of the most beautiful views I have ever seen.

By the end of day one, we're a mile high. The altitude is beginning to affect us now, although very slowly. Each step is a little harder, and each foot we climb is a bit more strenuous.

Laxmi cheerily announces that we would be going down two times today. "But then we have to go up. Steeeeeep up."

I thought descending would be a respite from the challenge of climbing. I was wrong. Sure, it's much easier on the breath, but the descents into the valleys are so steep, you can't lose your concentration for a second. Every step must be carefully planned, or you risk tumbling forward.

The ascents up the far sides of the valleys are brutal. Hundreds of uneven stairs that seem never-ending attack my legs, and my legs slowly relent under the pressure. By the end of day two, I am once again exhausted, though I'm lucky enough to avoid cramps. Stretching at night and in the morning makes me feel old, but it becomes a part of the routine.

We relax in the evenings, sharing tea and swapping stories between us. We toss casual questions back and forth. What's America like? How do you enjoy being a guide? One question at a time, we become friends and then family, going through the trek together.

On our second night, the guest house in Chomrong that promises electricity and Wi-Fi has neither. We have a romantic dinner, with a single candle serving as our only source of light and heat. It's too dark to notice the clouds that are creeping into the Annapurna range, but the sound of rain late at night is unmistakable.

We set off on our third day in heavy rain that shows no signs of letting up. I hike with my hood down. The rain on my forehead feels refreshing and keeps me cool. Underneath, I know I'm soaked. At some point, every piece of waterproof gear gives out when it's subjected to too much precipitation. Water has gotten through my pants, my shoes, my jacket, and my bag. I can stay warm as long as we keep moving, but when we stop for lunch, I'm freezing.

Guest houses are notoriously poorly insulated, so the temperature outside is the temperature inside. As we drink our tea and eat our lunch, the rain changes to what TV meteorologists would call a wintry mix. Once we start hiking again, it doesn't take long for it to switch to pure snow. It is now officially freezing outside, and the snow is piling up fast.

Farther up the trail, conditions are even worse. Hikers a day ahead of us are forced to wait out the weather, or worse, turn back. We're not that high yet, but we're getting close.

As long as we're moving, though, our surroundings are absolutely beautiful. A layer of snow blankets the ground and the trees. We may have missed a white Christmas in Bethlehem, but we are rewarded with a winter wonderland here. Occasionally, a break in the clouds lets us see the Himalayan peaks around us, soaring skyward. At the beginning of the hike, they seemed impossible to reach. Now they look to be just a few miles away.

This is my favorite stretch of the hike. Snow falling, boots crunching on fresh snow, all of us moving quietly. It's hard work, but it's enjoyable work. The air tastes cold and crisp, and my breath creates small wisps of condensation in the chill air. It is absolutely awesome. I feel alive in ways that I have rarely felt before.

We reach our guest house in Dovan as the sun sets. No amount of hiking would keep us truly warm with wet gear and no sun. Laxmi promises us a sort of heater at our guest house. The owners set up kerosene heaters in a pit under the table, which give visitors a chance to get warm and dry their clothing, two things we desperately need.

For some reason, the owners of the guest house refuse to fire up the heaters. At first, they claim that ten people have to be willing to pay for the heat (which cost 100 Nepali rupees, or almost exactly one US dollar), but when it becomes clear that every single person in the guest house wants heat, they claim the heaters are broken, much like the meters in Indian taxis that are always rumored to be broken when foreigners step in.

Our fourth day of hiking turns out to be beautiful weather. The sun is out, the weather is perfect, and the snow along the path is stunning. It feels good to keep moving, even as we cross the ten-thousand-feet mark. The altitude is affecting us, but we keep up a steady pace as we ascend ever higher.

A few times an hour, we pass hikers on their way down or porters carrying supplies from one village to another. They always greet us with a friendly *"Namaste!"* which means *a blessing upon you* in Nepali. Each time I exchange a *namaste* with a fellow trekker, I feel a bit more invigorated and a bit less tired. Knowing that we share something with others on the path makes me feel welcome in the Himalayas, even though I am farther from home than I have ever been.

Our goal on day four is Machapuchare Base Camp, colloquially called MBC. It is the final stop before Annapurna Base Camp. The two camps are separated by two hours of hiking and 1,500 feet. More importantly, MBC has electricity. ABC does not. We stay at MBC, where, this time, they fire up the under-the-table heaters, for which I am eternally grateful. The night is absolutely freezing, and the fifteen or so guests at the lodge huddle together as long as possible in the dining room. Temperatures drop so low that all the pipes freeze in the guest house. They send a porter down to the river to bring water for food and drinks.

We spend most of the evening in the small dining room, crowded around the table with a mix of hikers, guides, and porters. Anyone who forgets to close the outside door when coming into the dining room suddenly finds himself on the receiving end of a barrage of verbal lashes from everyone huddled inside. Two German teenagers sit across from us, sipping tea from an insulated metal container, bundled up in yak wool sweaters that I'm sure they bought for four dollars at a local stand before the hike. The conversation is fun and distracts us from the cold until we start telling stories about growing up in the States.

"You remember life before the Internet?" says one of the teenagers, apparently astonished that someone so old could be alive today.

I have never been so tempted to punch someone I just met. Or curl up in a ball and wallow in my own aging misery. I describe to them an era they've never experienced. Remembering phone numbers and sending letters to pen pals and relying on dial-up modems.

"Do you recognize this sound? *EEEEEeeeeeooooowwwwwooowoow*," I screech, imitating the sound of my old 14.4k modem.

"No, I have no idea what that is."

Now I understand why this hike is so exhausting. I'm apparently a dinosaur on the trail, a *Tyrannosaurus rex* only inches away from the hot tar pits of extinction.

With the temperature well below freezing and darkness already covering MBC, we call it a night. Our plan is simple. We will wake up early in the morning to make a push to ABC, where we can celebrate and have breakfast. Then we will begin our descent.

Cassie and I barely sleep. We're definitely excited, but that has nothing to do with our fitful rest. At twelve thousand feet, our bodies need more time to adjust to the elevation. The thin air keeps us from fully relaxing at night. I wake up more than once with my heart racing, trying to get enough oxygen to pump through my veins. We both sleep in our thermals and our sleeping bags, yet we're still bitterly cold all night.

We sleep through Cassie's alarm at 4:45 in the morning (I had set mine for 4:45 p.m. by accident). Laxmi wakes us up at 6:00 a.m. and tells us to hurry up. We leave most of our gear in the room. Tulasi will wait at MBC for us. This is a quick push to the top, and then we come right back down. Unfortunately, there will be nothing quick about the next three hours for me.

Only a handful of people have scaled Mount Everest in winter, and for good reason. Hurricane-force winds lash the world's highest peak, while freezing temperatures blanket anything above ten thousand feet. Weather in the Himalayas changes mercilessly during the coldest months, often shifting from bad to good to bad again within minutes.

At 13,500 feet, ABC isn't nearly as high as the tallest mountain on earth. But for a lowlander like me who grew up at sea level spending summers at the Jersey Shore, it is far outside of my comfort zone.

We filled our water bottles last night, but in the freezing temperatures of the final push, the water becomes ice. The sun isn't up yet, so there is nothing producing warmth, and I'm not moving fast enough to generate any significant amount of body heat. In these conditions, I learn what it means to suffer from exhaustion. The trek has drained every ounce of energy. I run out of gas and start running on fumes. Then I run out of those too.

Someone had written 1 HOUR TO ABC on a boulder along the way. I choke down some Oreo cookies and a few mouthfuls of water to keep me moving.

I know it'll take longer than the predicted hour, but a few minutes later I get exactly what I need. We see ABC in front of us. I know it's not close, and I know it will be hell to reach, but I have a visual goal. Finally, I begin to believe.

About thirty meters short of ABC, there is a sign welcoming us to Annapurna Base Camp. Only a final set of steps separates us from our goal. Cassie and Laxmi wait for me there, eager to take a picture of the three of us.

Cassie switches to her adorable falsetto voice that usually makes me smile. "Stop for a picture, babe!"

I'm too exhausted to smile and too close to stop. I snap at Cassie, "We're not there yet," and keep walking. She gets a picture of my back as I walk under the sign. Laxmi tells her we'll take pictures on the way down, which I think is the right idea.

I don't really remember the final few steps. I know they're hard, and I know I'm beyond tired, but I push through them as I have every other step on this final climb—one foot at a time. When I get to the top, I order the most expensive can of Coke I've ever had, sit down, and sip it very slowly. The sun is out, and it begins to warm everything up a bit.

I understand exactly what Sir Edmund Hillary meant when he became the first person to scale Everest in 1953. He said, "My first sensation was one of relief—relief that the long grind was over."

My accomplishment is in no way as significant, and I am at less than half of Hillary's final altitude. But I am relieved. Annapurna Base Camp sits in the middle of the Annapurna range, and the view while we relax for breakfast is like nothing I have ever seen before. Some of the highest mountains in the world arch toward the heavens around us. The snow makes everything bright and beautiful. We have reached our incredible destination, and we take our time this morning letting it soak in. The view around us. The climb we've just completed. And the sense of accomplishment we feel. There aren't many moments that I would describe as perfect. This is one of those moments.

Cassie and I order hot tea and breakfast while Laxmi hands us each a chocolate bar that he's been carrying to celebrate our final ascent. We all eat slowly, relishing the accomplishment of our bodies and, more important, our willpower. Every difficult step, every moment of exhaustion, every second of labor was absolutely worth it. We have reached ABC in winter through heavy snow. We have made it.

However, standing at 13,500 feet, having gone through the most phys-ically demanding experience of my life, I can't help but think that I'm only halfway done. Now I have to get back down. We hang out at ABC for about ninety minutes, snapping pictures and laughing toward the heavens before we start down. The sun is out, and it doesn't take much walking before we're nice and warm. As we pass the ABC sign, I yell a primal vic-tory scream as loud as I can and listen to it echo off the distant mountains for a long second. It feels right, and I sincerely apologize if I crushed any trekkers with an ensuing avalanche.

I had struggled to get all the way to ABC. Now I struggle to slow down. I want to run as fast as I can toward thicker air, warmer weather, and hot showers. On the snowy trail, I fall more than a few times into a pile of fresh Himalayan snow. In the elation of the post-ABC moment, I couldn't care less. I have made it to ABC, and I am ecstatic.

We have lunch at MBC on our way down, allowing some time for our gear to dry in the sun. Tulasi is waiting for us at MBC, and we laugh and hug after coming down from the top. Then we put on our gear, turn our back on this tiny little camp high in the Himalayas, and keep descending. On our way up, we pushed through rain, snow, and ice. Now all of that seems to vanish. The trails are mostly clear, the sun is out, and we're moving well, flying down the mountain at a fast but easy pace. There is a bounce in our step.

I don't know it yet, but I will pay dearly for what I have done to my body—the physical rigor and extreme stress I forced my system to endure. I have pushed my body to its absolute limit and beyond. For the last three or four weeks, my body had been breaking down slowly. The cramps on day one were evidence of these changes. Now I have passed the point of no return. The deterioration accelerates rapidly, and I am racing toward a physical and emotional judgment day.

Our descent back to our starting point proves far easier. Before we reached the top, we had, in a way, envied the climbers on their way down. They had conquered the challenge of ABC, celebrated, and could now breathe a bit easier as they descended. Now we were those trekkers, and groups of hikers on their way up asked us the same questions we had asked the trekkers before us. "Did you make it to the top?" "How was the view?" "How was the weather?" "Was it hard to get to ABC?"

The valleys that had been so hard to cross on the way up seem a little less steep and a little less difficult. The reward for reaching the top is a small town called Jhinu, another one of the guest house villages that exists specifically for trekkers. Only this one is special. Jhinu has natural hot springs nearby that are the perfect place to relax.

It takes us two days of trekking from ABC to reach Jhinu. We sleep in, savor a lazy breakfast, and eventually make our way down to the springs. They are as amazing as I imagined. Two different pools of wonderfully hot water sit next to the frigid Modi Khola river. The river itself is rough at this point, and the Himalayan water rushing over the rocks makes for a symphony of natural noise that fills the valley.

The hot springs melt away five days of hiking stress. We switch between the two pools—one is slightly hotter than the other—bathing in the warmth of the thermal waters. We spend three hours here. We could've spent three days.

Eventually, we leave Jhinu and the hot springs and keep descending toward what I consider a reasonable altitude to sustain life, specifically mine. We're ahead of schedule on our way down, so we only have to hike about three hours a day to finish on time. We eat long, lazy lunches and then longer, lazier dinners. We try different foods from the ubiquitous guest house menus, all of which taste almost exactly identical, no matter which town you're in, and all of which have been approved by something called the Sanctuary Tourism Entrepreneur Committee, which apparently gives cooking classes to Nepali guest house owners, given the ubiquity of the meals. We have Western pizzas that taste surprisingly . . . Western. We have Mexican burritos that taste surprisingly . . . Nepali. It doesn't matter. The food is great and we're all having a blast as we make our way through the final few towns of our trek.

On the morning of the eighth day, we reach Birethanti, one town away from where our hike had started. We take a picture of our family one more time and catch a cab to Pokhara. Our trek is over. We have made it up, and we have made it down.

In our own silly way, we are conquerors, vanquishing the challenge of this surreal hike. Looking back at pictures, it's almost impossible to imagine how difficult the hike was from MBC to ABC and how we made it all the way to the top. It's one of the most incredible memories of our travels so far.

Chapter 10

February 4, 2014
28°13'01.3"N 84°00'24.9"E
Matepani Gumba, Pokhara, Nepal

The problem with teaching English to young Buddhist monks in a hilltop monastery—and there is only one problem as far as I'm concerned—is the order in which you apply the modifiers *young* and *Buddhist*. We had assumed when we signed up for this stretch of volunteering that, above all else, our students would be monks. That is to say, we thought they would be quiet, meditative, diligent, and focused. To be fair, these stereotypes come from our assumptions about Buddhism and our preconceived notions about followers of the faith, of which we know little (and here I refer to both the faith and its followers). We believed monks would be willing students, great listeners, and eager participants in our classes. I am the teacher's assistant, ready to sharpen a pencil or enforce discipline as needed. Cassie is the teacher.

Our mistake is not that we were wrong about monks. We were wrong about our students. They aren't officially monks yet; they are monks-in-training, which means that, before they are officially monks, they are young—many of them not yet ten years old. They haven't mastered the peaceful, quiet demeanor that we normally associate with someone who has graduated to full monk and has devoted himself to a life of religious penitence and humility. Instead, they actively celebrate their abundance of adolescent energy, kicking and punching and disrupting their way through our classes in a way that reminds me a bit too much of myself, even if my elementary and middle school wardrobe involved fewer red robes and more sweatpants.

As monks-in-training, they will have the choice, upon turning eighteen, of becoming monks and devoting their life to the monastery and the religion or leaving the monastery and living what we would consider a normal life. From what I can understand, nearly every one becomes a monk. It's all they've ever known.

Put a bunch of these kids in a beautifully colorful and completely isolated monastery on top of a hill on the outskirts of Pokhara with no female influence whatsoever, and there you have Matepani Gumba, a home for exiled Tibetan monks living in Nepal. Kids who aren't in class scream and run amok in the exact way you'd expect from young children living in a giant dorm full of testosterone, a hormone these juveniles are just now discovering, though it is strictly forbidden to use said hormone, especially if that use is directed at a member of the opposite sex. Since the only such person within the immediate vicinity is my wife, I come to appreciate this moratorium on the use of testosterone quite a bit.

The students are a joy to work with, even if the classes are just a bit too long; everyone loses focus during the last few minutes. We spend the most time with our youngest students, some of whom have absolutely no understanding of the English language. My heart reaches out to these kids in particular, since I remember my first day of prekindergarten like it was yesterday. I sat in the sandbox and cried all day with my twin sister because we didn't speak a word of English. We had recently emigrated from Israel, and I spoke only Hebrew.

Cassie takes all of our students through the alphabet and the days of the week and the months of the year every morning, mixing in questions about the weather and the temperature. It's awesome to watch her in her element, because it doesn't take long to see real progress with our students. I call them our students, but they are very much her students, and everything they learn is a consequence of her instruction, not my pencil sharpening.

There are four levels of English classes that are numbered Levels 1, 2, 4, and 6. I can't for the life of me fathom what Buddhists have against the first two odd prime numbers, but there is no such thing as Level 3 or Level 5. And if that makes no sense, the monastery's system of placing students in each level is completely ridiculous. They are placed in their English level based on how proficient they are at Tibetan, with the unfortunate consequence that a student who is phenomenal at English but awful at Tibetan will be in the same class as a student who has no aptitude for languages and is bad at both. That's like placing me in a mechanical engineering class based on how well I performed in underwater basket weaving.

Every morning, we wake up and begin the one-hour walk to Matepani Gumba. We could take a bus to a major bus park and another bus to the monastery, but we enjoy the morning and afternoon walks, since it gives us a front row seat to the daily insanity that is driving in Nepal. Far too many cars fill far too small a road, and the only thing that determines who gets to go where, as far as I can tell, is who has the loudest car horn and how vigorously he employs it.

This is the great urban symphony that we enjoy during our walk. As we near our destination, we have one final test to overcome. Matepani Gumba sits on top of a hill, and we have to climb three hundred steps before we can officially say, "We made it." The monastery itself is breathtaking, and we feel privileged to see it every day. It is enclosed within a bright orange wall. Much like the great facade of Petra, you don't see it until you round the final turn through the gate. The monastery is an explosion of intense oranges and reds and greens and blues, each detail intricately painted as if to maximize the aesthetic value of the monastery. A row of columns supports the front of the building. At their base, the columns are a rich red with carved yellow stripes, but as they climb, they switch to a meticulous multicolor design that wraps around the entire building. As you go even higher, the colors switch to a green, blue, and flowered pattern on the window shutters before changing once again to red. On top of the monastery is a bright golden statue that looks like two resting deer staring at a golden wheel. That statue symbolizes the wheels of life and time, the fruits of abundance, and so much more than I understand. The walls on the inside of the building feature beautiful paintings telling the story of Buddha. A big courtyard dominates the space in front of the square monastery, and we often see prayer groups gathering here. The courtyard of the monastery provides a stunning view of the Annapurna range in the distance. On clear days—of which there are many—the snow-covered mountains fill the horizon, almost as if jostling for space in your field of vision. I look out at those mountains and remember our incredible hike, which already feels like a barely perceptible dream.

Only once did we ever spot a Westerner at the monastery. She came in to take some pictures and was gone before we exchanged pleasantries.

Matepani Gumba feels like our little secret, even if it is the most famous monastery in Pokhara.

Rows of small dorms surround the main prayer building. Our classrooms are in the same buildings as the dorms, and we show up a few minutes early every day to set up our lessons. Above all else, our students are fun. They may have some trouble focusing, and they steal one another's pencils and notebooks in ways that I imagine Buddha would frown upon, but they're eager to learn and they love trying to impress Cassie. Without conducting a deeper psychoanalysis, I think they like having a woman around. When Cassie asks a question, every hand darts up and the students yell, "Miss! Miss! Miss!" since they can't pronounce the "z" sound in "Ms! Ms! Ms!" Their willingness to volunteer has nothing to do with their knowledge of the answer, since they exhibit plenty of the former and none of the latter. They just want the teacher's attention. When we start teaching them to name fruits using a set of flashcards, every student inevitably yells out "Cherry!" when we flip the first card, regardless of what fruit the card actually displays.

We teach two classes in the morning, then have lunch with our students, which is always some variation of dahl bat. Dahl bat is the most common Nepali food, consisting of lentils, beans, and rice. For lunch and dinner every day, we eat dahl bat, sometimes even for breakfast. The curry flavor mixed in with the lentil soup is very palatable, even if it becomes somewhat monotonous by the eighty-seventh time we have the same meal. Our students politely bring us refills of water and second helpings of rice, and they clean our plates for us when we finish eating.

On one particularly beautiful afternoon, the monks invite us to have some tea before our walk home. We gladly accept their hospitality, and they pour us each a cup of their brew. According to the canister, we will be drinking Tibetan salt tea. I'm always excited to try new foods and drinks, especially if they're from a new culture or region. I eagerly take my first sip of this mysterious beverage.

Generally, I find it incredibly impolite to vomit in front of or on a monk, but Tibetan salt tea is so horrifically awful that I weigh the pros and cons. Pros: I no longer have to have this drink in my mouth. Cons: I may be summarily kicked out of the monastery. It's a difficult decision. The liquid in my cup—if you can call it a liquid, since it's much thicker than normal tea—is yellow and viscous. It looks and tastes exactly like melting a stick of salted butter and serving it as a refreshment. Why on earth would you do this? I have no idea, but it's a very popular drink among monks. Our students apparently drink it every day at tea time. Cassie takes one sip and hands me the rest of her cup. It would be impolite not to finish the drink—not as impolite as throwing up on a monk, but still undesirable enough—so I now have to consume both cups of tea, which requires a not inconsiderable amount of gastrointestinal and testicular fortitude.

After lunch, we have one more class to teach before heading to our host family's house.

Krishna and Bimala's house is a three-story concrete building in the northern part of the city. They rent out the first floor, live on the second floor, and have rooms for the volunteers on the third floor. That's where we stay. Our room is spartan by any standards. We have two small beds in our room, so Cassie and I sleep separately every night. Our backpacks and clothing sit in two piles in the corner adjacent to the door. The bathroom is one door over, and we share it with the other volunteers.

Bimala wakes us up every morning with a hot cup of tea or coffee. Most mornings, we are already awake because the neighbor's rooster shrieks bloody murder at four o'clock sharp. I wish no ill will on anyone or anything, man or beast, but I come to hate that rooster with every ounce of my being, even more than the local stray dogs that host their own bona fide Wrestlemania event early every morning and twice on Thursdays. By the time we come down to the kitchen, Bimala has breakfast ready, which is either dahl bat or oatmeal. We normally don't see Krishna until dinner, since he teaches at a local school and runs the Alliance Nepal volunteer organization. Bimala is a stay-at-home mom, a task that becomes infinitely more difficult and time-consuming without modern appliances. She cooks, cleans, and does laundry by hand every day, and she does it all with a perpetual smile.

Krishna and Bimala become our second family. We have dinner with them every weeknight, where we tell them about our students and our classes. After dinner, we hang out with their two kids and their nephew in the living room, playing word games to improve their English. Their nephew's family lives in rural Nepal, where quality schools are hard to find, so the family sent him to live with Krishna and Bimala so he could get a better education. Krishna's dream is for his children to attend college in America, and he makes them complete their homework before they can goof off.

We spend weekends at Lakeside, where we pay two dollars to do our laundry once a week and I splurge on my weekly shave, which sets me back three dollars. We always stay at the same hotel, paying ten dollars a night for a room.

On our last weekend in Pokhara, we take a boat across Phewa Lake to the World Peace Stupa, a beautiful white pagoda that sits atop a mountain overlooking Pokhara and the lake. The hike up the mountain takes forty-five minutes, and I feel completely wiped out when we reach the top. A sign explaining the history of the World Peace Stupa informs us that this is one of eighty Peace Pagodas around the globe, which I find incredible, since I've never heard of the other seventy-nine.

As we walk around the stupa, I confide in Cassie something that's been on my mind lately.

"I'm sick and tired of being sick and tired," I tell her, choking back tears. Recently, we've both noticed that I've lost a bit of weight. My arms and legs have become rail thin, and both of our parents asked if I was on a diet the last time we Skyped with them. I've also been feeling weak, and it has gotten worse since our Himalayas hike. We talk about a few options—going to a doctor, calling doctors back home, visiting a hospital—but we decide the first step is to figure out how much weight I've lost.

We find a pharmacy in Lakeside that lets us use their scale for a second. I step onto the scale, but the number staring back at me doesn't make any sense.

"Are you sure this scale is right?" I ask the woman behind the counter.

"Yes," she says, smiling back at me.

I start converting kilograms to pounds in my head. Multiply by two. Figure out ten percent, then add that twice. That means I weigh . . . wait, double check the number . . . 180 pounds? If that's right, I have lost forty-five pounds. I thought I had lost twenty pounds at most, but forty-five means I have lost nearly a quarter of my body weight from my usual 225. How is that even possible?

Lacking anything that would qualify as helpful medical knowledge, we email some of my doctor friends back home and describe my symptoms. Weight loss. Thirst. A constant need to pee. Weakness. We even Skype with one of them so that she can see me, or at least a pixelated version of me, which is the best we can manage over Nepali Wi-Fi. Their verdict is unanimous: malnutrition. Since entering Nepal, I have been on a vegetarian diet, eating far fewer calories than I normally eat since there isn't too much junk food here. The massive infusion of rice into my diet explains the thirst, since rice can draw fluids out of the system. And the weakness and weight loss come from a lack of protein. All I have to do is eat more. One of my friends says I have the classic symptoms of diabetes, but we both agree that's incredibly unlikely, since there is no history of diabetes in my family.

Back at Krishna and Bimala's house, we email the medical update to my family. We didn't want to consult them first because we suspected they would immediately and irreversibly freak out. We were right. They start sending panicked emails, begging me to go to the doctor. On a Skype call with my parents at night, I make a simple deal with them. I'll go to the doctor if they track their diet and go to a personal trainer. My parents are overweight and putting on more pounds. In Israel, a friend of the family had told me to force them to get help. Now, I use their concerns about my health as leverage for my worries about theirs.

"Not even the Jews in Auschwitz lost weight as fast as you," my dad says. "You have to go to a doctor."

"I'll go to a doctor when you see a personal trainer."

"What does our weight have to do with your health?"

"You can't worry about my health until you take care of your own. Write down what you eat for three straight days and see a personal trainer."

"You're not going to survive that long, and I'm not coming to Nepal to bury you."

"Okay then. I'll try to die in Laos so you can at least visit somewhere you've never been for my funeral."

The conversation goes around in circles, each of us trying to get the other to seek help. But each circle becomes more frustrating, and our voices rise in unison until we're yelling at one another. My mom starts crying, which makes me feel worse than I already do. I refuse to find a doctor because they refuse to see a personal trainer. And we have too much on our agenda coming up. We have one more week of volunteering before we return to Thailand for scuba lessons and the continuation of our Southeast Asia explorations. I promise to find a doctor when we have some free time in Thailand. By the time we hang up, I am furious at my parents, and I suspect they feel much the same way toward me.

When we arrive at the monastery for our final week of teaching, one of the workers kindly informs us that the monastery has announced a holy day, called a *pooja*, and canceled morning classes. There will be one class in the afternoon. We can sit around the monastery for five hours and wait for class or we can simply come back tomorrow. Cassie and I decide to take advantage of the unexpected free day to visit a doctor.

We hail a cab to Quality Healthcare, one of the few medical providers in Pokhara and one of even fewer that has any positive reviews online. We walk in and take a seat in the waiting room. The doctor's assistant invites us into the examination room a moment later.

A doctor, whom I'll call Dr. Griffiths, introduces himself. "What seems to be the problem?" I describe my symptoms to Dr. Griffiths. He doesn't look right at me, instead tilting his head ever so slightly to his left in a way that comes across as mildly disconcerting, as if he's not quite listening to me. I suspect this is how he focuses, picturing my symptoms in his mind, but it would be a bit more reassuring if he occasionally turned to glance in my direction.

The doctor has his assistant take my temperature and blood pressure. He says I have a low-grade fever, and he comes to the same conclusion every other doctor has, that I've been suffering from malnutrition since coming to Nepal. What I need, he says, is some protein and vitamins. He recommends juices and chicken, and sends me on my way.

"Don't you want to take a blood test?" I ask.

"I can if you want me to."

"I want you to."

The blood test reveals that I am healthy, although with a minor infection. Dr. Griffiths gives me a multivitamin, electrolyte powder packets, and an antibiotic for the infection.

I can't wait to get home and email my family. I was right all along, as backed up by the opinions of five different doctors now. Cassie and I stop at the store to pick up some extra nutrition—pomegranate juice, soy milk, and a few other snacks. Up in our room, I compose an email that I hope will silence the insanity, liberally adding my own sarcastic annoyance to the mix.

Mon, Feb 10, 2014 at 7:01 a.m.
Oren Liebermann
To: Yaffa Liebermann, Eli Liebermann, Tamar Brooks, Hadas Liebermann

Subject: You should all convert to Buddhism

I had promised all of you that I would go get a blood test when we had a free day in Thailand in a week. This morning, we went to volunteer at our monastery, only to find out that Buddhists had decided to schedule an unannounced day of prayer and canceled class.

Given the free day, we went to a medical clinic, got a blood test, and saw a doctor. As we expected, the blood test showed no infection, no illness, and nothing unhealthy. Dad's doomsday prognostications of my imminent death were absolute bullshit, which we all should've have recognized immediately. (Don't worry, apology accepted.)

The doctor gave me electrolyte powder, because he agreed my diet lacks nutrients. He recommended eggs, fresh fruits, and lots of fluids. He also gave me a pill for worms. He said worms can have no symptoms, but can suck nutrients away from the body. That's a one-time pill that I take in a few hours. He said there's no way to know if it's worms, but it's fairly common here and the pill has no side effects.

In 3 days, we'll find out if there's any bacteria or a parasite in my blood, but he said there's no way that's the case since I have no stomach pain, nausea, or diarrhea.

I will go to him again on Friday to check my weight and see if anything has changed.

Let me be clear about one thing. The mass paranoia and hysteria on that side of the Atlantic was absolutely unacceptable. Tamar and Erez started with reasonable emails, then went into freak-out mode when Mom chimed in. Our health is our number one concern, and we take care of ourselves and each other. Your sharing bullet points and sending childish, guilt-trip emails (most of which got snide responses or automatic deletions) were patently ridiculous. You're thousands of miles away, and when I tell you that I've described my symptoms to doctors with valid medical opinions, I expect you to respect those opinions instead of voicing your own wild guesses about what's going on. (Mom calling my in-laws was particularly outrageous.)

We learned that what was wrong was exactly what our doctors told us (and what we told you in the first email, in case you forgot)—a lack of nutrients and a low-calorie diet for too long. We've made the adjustments to my diet and I will be fine (again, as I told you in the first email, in case you forgot).

Now that you're done worrying about my health, you can make sure the parents fill out their 3-day food log and meet with my nutritionist/personal trainer.

You're welcome,
Oren

Improvement does not come quickly. The next morning, I'm feeling as bad, if not worse. On a one-hour walk to the monastery, I drag my feet along the sidewalk. My mouth is half open as my breathing drags. I stare down at the street a few feet in front of me, barely able to muster enough energy to focus my eyes on one particular spot. At the bottom of the three hundred stairs to the monastery, I stop. For a long time, I stand still, trying to find the courage to attempt the first step. Once I start, I know I will have no choice but to keep climbing every single one of those steps, and that seems like a monumental task right now. I begin working my way up, trying to keep up some forward momentum with a slow rhythm. One step every two seconds.

Once at the top, I collapse onto a bench and polish off half my water bottle in one swig. I need to stop drinking for a moment only so I can swallow a few breaths before I continue. Then I start walking to the bathroom, knowing I will have to pee in a few minutes.

I tell Cassie I need to rest. I spend the entire first period sleeping in the library, trying to find the strength to help my wife teach.

I get through the next class but only manage to eat a few bites at lunch. I push my food around my plate, wondering if it will look any more tempting in a few minutes. My appetite is nearly gone, and my enthusiasm for the final group of the day goes with it. At one point, they're not responding to Cassie's request for silence. Without energy, my patience is nonexistent. I walk over to the nearest table and slam my fist down on the desk. I know I'm weak, but the noise is loud enough to shock the class into silence. As a teacher, I am a failure. But as a disciplinarian, I'm showing some real promise.

At night, I notice a strange taste at the back of my mouth. Almost a fruity taste that won't go away. I'm sure it's the aftertaste of the electrolyte powder, which has an orange flavor much akin to an awful spin-off of orange Gatorade. But when I sip the electrolyte water, it's obvious that it's an entirely different flavor. Whatever is creating the taste at the back of my mouth is something different, and it won't go away, no matter how many times I rinse out my mouth.

The next day is the same. I have to rest through the first class, I barely eat anything at lunch, and I struggle through the rest of the day. Even the students take notice.

"Are you okay?"

"No." I don't even bother feigning health.

"Oren is very sick," Cassie says from the front of class. She has no idea how right she is.

Chapter 11

February 13, 2014
28°14'13.4"N 83°58'44.8"E
Lakeside, Pokhara, Nepal

I wake up feeling sapped of all my energy, completely exhausted to my very core. All week I had felt tired, and the creeping lethargy has only gotten worse in the last forty-eight hours. On Tuesday and Wednesday, I had made it to Matepani Gumba only to pass out in the library during the first class I was supposed to teach with Cassie. The hour walk to and from the monastery feels like running a marathon, and the three hundred stairs to the top might as well have been the Hawaii Ironman.

During meals, I force myself to eat as much as I can per the doctor's orders. But I can scarcely down a few bites. For the first time in our relationship, Cassie eats more than I do. Far more. It's not a function of her appetite dramatically increasing but of mine effectively disappearing. Food doesn't look appealing to me anymore, and I want to retch with each new serving of dal bhat placed in front of me. The lentils, beans, and rice that are the staple of every Nepali meal look absolutely abhorrent to me, even though as recently as last week I was having second helpings.

I try to get my nutrition through juices and soy milk, drinking mouthfuls each morning and evening to sate my unquenchable thirst. After waking up, I double-fist pomegranate juice and soy milk, alternating between the two cardboard containers. I also manage to swallow a few small bananas and oranges throughout the day. But each spoonful of rice and each forkload of curry require a cup of water to swallow. In the morning, Bimala's oatmeal only goes down with equal parts water and nausea.

At dinner the night before, I ate only a few bites. Krishna and Bimala both said I didn't look very good, so Cassie and I agreed it was time to go back to the doctor. She would teach, and I would try to figure out what was wrong with me.

But first I have to summon the energy to get out of bed. For ten minutes, I sit on the narrow wooden frame, hunched over on the thin pad that hardly qualifies as a mattress, unmoving with my elbows on my knees, resting my head in my hands. All I have to do is straighten my legs, tilt my back, lean forward, and stand up. And that seems impossible. I am somehow more tired now than I was before I went to bed.

Eventually, I realize that sitting on my bed on the third floor of a house in Pokhara, Nepal, isn't getting me any closer to the doctor, and it's certainly not making me any better. Bimala brings up some coffee, and a short time later, I walk the quarter mile to the main road where I can grab a taxi to the doctor's office.

Once again, Dr. Griffiths sees me moments after I walk in. This time, we sit and talk in what would qualify as the waiting room in any doctor's office that I've ever visited, except here, without anyone else in the building except Dr. Griffiths's assistant, it becomes a makeshift examination room.

"What seems to be the problem?" he says in his thick Indian accent, restarting the diagnostic conversation from the very beginning as if he hadn't just seen me earlier in the week. He is seated to my right, and we are halfway between looking at each other and looking at the wall in front of us.

"I'm just not feeling better. I'm feeling a lot worse." I tell him about the last couple of days, eating more food, drinking more juice, finding fresh fruit—following his instructions exactly. "And it doesn't seem to be working."

I tell him I have all the same symptoms: parched mouth, never-ending thirst, a constant need to urinate, and an awful taste at the back of my throat. Oh, and one more.

"I haven't . . ." I pause, seeking the right words. "I haven't gone to the bathroom in five days." I hope it comes out eloquently, but in my state of exhaustion, the higher rules of general etiquette no longer qualify as important or even relevant.

Dr. Griffiths nods to his assistant, who knows exactly what to get and where to find it. I have the distinct impression that Dr. Griffiths talked about my possible return to his assistant, and they both knew what to do in the event that I found myself in the Quality Healthcare office once again.

The doctor opens a small black case, about half the size of my old lunch box, and pulls out a navy blue medical device shaped like a deformed oval. I recognize it immediately as a blood sugar monitor, having seen some of my friends test their blood sugar when I was a kid.

Dr. Griffiths's assistant, who has been nothing but helpful since we first met him on Monday, pricks my finger and draws a tiny bead of blood that sits ever so gently on the tip of my extended digit. He scoops up the drop-let with the tip of what looks like a small plastic strip and inserts it into the monitor. I watch the numbers blink on the monochrome display.

5 . . . 4 . . . 3 . . . 2 . . . 1 . . . 406.

The doctor takes a deep breath. Whatever he's gleaned from the num-ber does not bode well for me, though I have no idea what it means. There is a moment's hesitation that I will never forget, a well-defined temporal demarcation that denotes the end of one era of my life and the beginning of another. This brief second is the present, and it sharply separates the past and the future.

"I'm sorry to tell you, my friend," Dr. Griffiths says, pausing mid-sentence, "but you are a diabetic."

He allows the weight of the news to sink in. In the brief span of one compound sentence, my life, my health, and my well-being have been twisted, warped, deformed into something completely different. If I'm breathing, I'm unaware of it. If I'm thinking, it's not in coherent thoughts. Mere spasms of syllables and phrases echo off of the suddenly empty walls of my mind.

Holy shit.

I'll say that again.

Holy shit.

A few of the doctors I had spoken with back in the States earlier in the week mentioned there was an outside chance that I have diabetes, but they didn't believe it, and neither did I. One does not "catch" diabetes in the same way that one catches a cold or a flu. My whole body goes numb, and so does my mind. I cannot think. I cannot feel. I cannot reason. I can barely talk. Oxygen, which, until this very moment, constituted about 20 percent of the air around me, suddenly seems overtly and conspicuously lacking.

There is an awkward silence that I'm sure everyone who has gone through a life-changing diagnosis would recognize immediately.

"I am diabetic too, and you will be okay," the doctor reassures me.

Somewhere in the deepest parts of my subconscious, I know what he says is right. It must be right. I have friends who have diabetes, and they're doing great. But in this first minute, it's impossible to believe.

I feel like I got kicked in the nuts. Swiftly, solidly, and squarely in the jewels of my masculine plumbing. Except that's more of a physical sensation, and this is almost entirely emotional. I think the physical pain of getting crushed in the testicles would actually soften the emotional shock of such an unlikely diagnosis. I firmly believe that doctors should keep a small but well-trained staff of short people around to kick patients in the nuts before major diagnoses to soften the second blow by focusing on the first.

"Okay," I say with as much mirth as I can muster, which amounts to a whopping sum of barely none. My plans to keep traveling—to get on board a plane to Thailand, to ride a train to Koh Tao, to earn my scuba certificate—have vanished. Instead, I have one simple mission that is now the focus of every bit of my energy. I need to go home.

Doctor Griffiths explains to me that I have late-diagnosis type 1 diabetes. In short, I am thirty-one years old with juvenile diabetes. Of course, this doesn't really mean anything to me, but, from what I can understand from his explanations, my diagnosis at this stage of life is astronomically rare.

But regardless of the minuscule percentage of people diagnosed later in life with type 1 diabetes, 100 percent of me is diagnosed, and, at this moment, that's all I care about.

"Doctor, I will book tickets to go home as soon as possible to get more medical help. Am I okay to fly home?"

"Yes, you will be fine. Just make sure to drink lots of water. Go to a doctor as soon as you get home."

The appointment ends a few minutes later. He asks me to come back the following morning before breakfast to test my blood sugar two more times. He wants to do a fasting blood sugar test, which he explains is a test on an empty stomach that measures my baseline blood sugar after not eating. It is one of the first tests used to determine if someone has diabetes or prediabetes. Then he wants me to eat breakfast and return exactly two hours later for a postprandial blood sugar test that will show how my body handles sugars and how much insulin my pancreas is producing.

I thank him for his help and promise to return early in the morning.

I don't remember anything from the walk to the taxi stand or the cab ride home. I know I have to get in touch with Cassie at the monastery and tell her to come home now. We only have one more day of teaching left, but neither of us will be able to attend those classes. We won't be able to say goodbye to the kids we have worked with for three weeks, and I know that will upset Cassie. These are more than her students; they are her classroom children, and she cares for each and every one of them.

On the way home, I run over a mental checklist of things I need to do. I have to talk to my parents. I have to talk to Mark, a missionary doctor in Kathmandu whom Cassie's family church supports. I have to talk to my host family. And I have to talk to Drew, my friend who has had diabetes since he was ten years old. He is perpetually optimistic, and I need an injection of his positive attitude almost as much as I need an injection of insulin.

I make my way up to the front door of our home and knock. Bimala answers.

"Please have Krishna call the monastery to tell Cassie to come home immediately," I say to Bimala. Or at least that's what I plan on saying, but the words don't come out. I had rehearsed the sentence a dozen times in the cab, compartmentalized the thirteen words in my mind so that they're parked at the proverbial tip of my tongue, but I am suddenly and completely incapable of coherent speech.

The second I see Bimala, I break down in tears. Heaving sobs wrack my entire body. My arms hang limply by my sides, and my chin falls down to my chest. I have lost forty-five pounds—I am lighter than I've been since high school—yet my legs feel like they're supporting a metric ton. The diagnosis that seemed surreal at the doctor's office becomes very real in an instant.

Each time I try to form a sentence—to tell Bimala to call Krishna, to take the first steps toward the Western hemisphere—my tongue fails me. I want desperately to be home, to be away from this moment and this disease; I want Cassie right next to me, but I can't formulate any of that into words.

Bimala comes over to me immediately and hugs me. She stops being a mother and becomes *my* mother. I am nearly ten thousand miles away from my family, and she knows intuitively that I need support. In her arms, I don't try to hold back the tears. There's no point. They completely overpower me.

More than a few minutes pass before I finally vocalize the sentence I've been trying to say since I walked in the door. She calls Krishna immediately, and Cassie is on her way home a few minutes later.

Up in our room, I try to gather my thoughts, but the whole world seems too out of focus. There is no calm. There is no order. Everywhere I look and everything I feel is chaos. I know I have to call my folks, but I want Cassie with me first. I know I should book tickets home, but I need Cassie's help. My hands are shaking too much to be of any use.

Everything makes sense and nothing makes sense. I begin to understand why I've been tired for two months, why I almost collapsed near Annapurna Base Camp, why I've been so thirsty, why I lost my appetite. All sorts of "what happened" questions suddenly have an answer. Yet I can't understand much simpler questions, the ones without qualifiers or specifics. Why? And how?

Stripped of all the other details and circumstances, these are the questions I need answered. And yet I feel that these answers are farther away than my home. The latter is a few plane rides away. The former has no such roadmap, no easy-to-follow directions to comprehension.

Sitting on Cassie's bed, staring at my computer screen and wondering what to do next, I am able to control my breathing, but only for a moment. As soon as Cassie walks in the door, I break down again and hug her. For the last few weeks, I have been physically weak. Now I am emotionally drained too. Nothing in my thirty-one years has prepared me for this, and it shatters my suddenly tenuous grip on this world.

When I am calm enough to speak in full sentences, I call home, where it is 2:30 in the morning. Last week, Krishna installed a small solar panel for his Wi-Fi router so he could have Internet all day. That small investment allows me to call home immediately instead of waiting for power to kick on at night. My mom answers the third time I call, unaccustomed to her phone ringing at this hour.

"Hallo?" She is groggy, wondering who is calling at this hour, not realizing yet that it's me.

"I'm so sorry, Ima. I went to the doctor again today because I was feeling worse. I found out I am diabetic." I pause so she can process what I just said. "You were right. I was wrong. I'm coming home."

I describe the morning's visit to the doctor in as much detail as I can remember while sitting in the stairwell near the router to make sure the connection doesn't drop. Cassie is already preparing our bags in our room.

"Oren, I'm glad you listened to your body and went back to the doctor."

"Is Aba there?"

"Aba is in Houston. You can call him now."

"Ima. I love you. I'll see you soon."

I call my dad a moment later. He answers on the first ring, still awake after a late business flight.

"Hi Aba. You can yell at me as much as you want now. You were right. I have a disease. I went back to the doctor today and found out I have diabetes." The words still seem strange coming from my mouth. I have *diabetes*.

But my dad doesn't yell. His words are calm and measured. "I'm happy that you went to the doctor. When will you be home?"

"We're gonna look at flights in a minute. We'll email you when we have flights booked."

Cassie and I sit down to look at flights. First, we need an early afternoon flight to Kathmandu, which Krishna books for us. Then, we need a flight home. Apparently, a Kathmandu–New York flight isn't exactly in high demand, so we'll have to connect somewhere. After a few minutes of searching, we book Qatar Airways Flight 651 from Kathmandu to Doha. The flight leaves tomorrow night and arrives in Qatar at midnight. After an eight-hour layover, we will fly from Doha to New York. If the flight schedule can be trusted, I will be on American soil at 2:05 p.m. and home from the airport ninety minutes later.

Normally, as someone with an Israeli name and Israeli visa stamps in my passport, connecting in the middle of an Arab country wouldn't be high on my to-do list, but geopolitical rivalries are of no consequence to me at the moment. I want to go home.

I need to go home.

We email the flight info to my family, and then I sit down to compose another email to my siblings.

Thu, Feb 13, 2014 at 2:48 a.m.
Oren Liebermann
To: Erez Liebermann, Tamar Brooks, Hadas Liebermann

Subject: *I have never been more wrong*

On Monday and Tuesday, the doctor said the only problem was lack of nutrients. I wasn't feeling any better, so I went back to the doctor today and he double-checked my blood sugar (which had been fine on Tuesday).

Today, my blood sugar came back 406 mg. A normal person's blood sugar is 150 mg. (Normal blood glucose ranges from 70 to 140 mg, but I didn't know it at the time.) *In short, it looks like I am diabetic. The doctor will test my blood sugar twice tomorrow, which will likely confirm the diagnosis.*

Then we're on our way home for as long as it takes for me to put on weight and get the meds I need.

I apologize to all of you for the massive attitude I gave you. I will apologize in person when I see you again. But we're Liebermanns—arguments are what we do.

We will see you all soon. It looks like we will get back Saturday afternoon. Erez—we'll probably stop by your house on the way home, and then you can drink Blue Label for me.

All the love in the world,
Oren and Cassie

I compose one more quick email to Drew. I already need his help and his optimism, even if he is halfway around the world. Though I am still unable to comprehend the last few hours, let alone the rest of my life, I know how helpful he would be, both in terms of his advice and his attitude.

Thu, Feb 13, 2014 at 2:50 a.m.
Oren Liebermann
To: Drew Greenspan

Subject: *I'm gonna need your help these next few weeks*

I was feeling awful for a few weeks here in Nepal. I finally went to the doctor and he checked my blood sugar. The test came back 406 mg. Looks like I'm diabetic, which we will confirm tomorrow. I'll let you know.

I'll be home in a couple of days—the right move seems to be coming home to recover, put on some weight, and learn how to use an insulin pump and do the shots and all that. We'll do dinner one night.

We start making preparations for the journey home. We pack up our clothing and get our bags ready to travel. We clean out our room, strip our beds, and throw out any leftover food we haven't eaten. I am able to put aside my perpetual exhaustion, knowing that I have precious few hours to get ready for an incredibly long and challenging journey back home and back to good health.

Throughout the afternoon and the evening, the tears keep coming. In powerful tides, the waves of heaving and sobbing ebb and flow. One moment I am fine, rolling up my spare pants to pack in the bottom of my backpack. Then I am gasping for air, searching for Cassie, for home, for help, for something stable upon which to right my violently yawing world.

Tamar is the first to respond. She's in Kenya, so while it's the middle of the night for most of my family, it's the middle of the day for her.

Thu, Feb 13, 2014 at 3:46 a.m.
Tamar Brooks
To: Oren Liebermann

Subject: RE: I have never been more wrong

Oren—
Mom just called me. I am heading home immediately to try to reach you. I wish you were right!!! I wish it was just food. But as I said, that is a massive weight loss in too short a period.

I am not a doctor nor ever claim to be, but I am not sure you can wait. Your body is probably producing ketones, and that is the problem. You need a hospital now and they need to flush you with IVs and meds. It is poison to your system. This is why you are so thirsty. Ketones smell and Cassie should be able to smell that you have a different odor. You cannot survive a flight like this. I am not kidding. I spent days in the hospital with Pam when she had this. She was diabetic.

Delhi and Singapore have good hospitals. We have money. Get to one of those now and get care.

Sincerely,
Tamar Brooks

I have no idea what she's referring to—ketones? poison? smell?—and I decide to ignore her advice, since I have the medical backing and sound advice of Dr. Griffiths, who cleared me to fly home. I kindly inform her that I'm not going to Delhi or Singapore for the simple reason that I'm coming home.

Drew responds a short time later. He is up early with his newborn, and I knew he would get back to me as soon as he checked his email.

Thu, Feb 13, 2014 at 5:03 a.m.
Drew Greenspan
To: Oren

Subject: RE: I'm gonna need your help these next few weeks

Oh man... that sucks but out of all the things to happen and go wrong this is by far the most manageable. we can handle this no problem.

First thing were gonna do is get together and figure out our plan. I would say nutritionist first to get a good baseline for diet. There where I'm falling apart lately ;) and honestly diet and exercise (and a little insulin of course) are by far most important.

How do you feel right now BTW? Are you on insulin now? Is there a chance that its a shrot term abbe ration? Its pretty late in the fame foe type 1 diabetes. Though if it is you need to talk to Sean B. He ended up with type 1 diabetes a few years bakc and he can prob offer SME gpod insights as to how he changed things life wise at this point.

you don't think tpy caught it from me during one of our long man hugs do you??

Where are you flying back to? And when?

Grammatical and typographical errors aside, Drew's email makes me smile for the first time all day. I never really expected that I would have to go through this alone, but Drew's help and positive outlook are already reassuring. I'm not even back in the States yet, and he is already my mentor.

We plan to be at the doctor's office early so we can confirm my diagnosis, run by the monastery to drop off some school supplies, take a quick shower, and catch our first of three flights home.

Logistically, it's a pain in the ass to get home from Pokhara. There are only three flights a day from Pokhara to Kathmandu. They're short flights—twenty-five minutes—but they all leave between one and five in the afternoon. If we can't find a late flight out of Kathmandu, we have to plan on spending the night in the Nepali capital, meaning we have to add twenty-four hours of travel to our itinerary. There are a few options home once we get to Kathmandu. We can go east through Hong Kong or west through the Middle East—Abu Dhabi, Dubai, or Doha. Each of these flight schedules has an eight- to ten-hour layover, so getting home will require a bare minimum of thirty hours of travel, starting with our first flight to Kathmandu.

It will be a busy day, but in the back of my mind, I know it's one step closer to getting treatment and going home. That bit of good news isn't bright enough to qualify as the light at the end of the tunnel, but it's all I've got at the moment.

When I had climbed out of bed this morning, everything seemed to make sense. Life fell into a neat, orderly routine of waking up, exploring, traveling, and going to sleep—or at least as neat and orderly as the travel lifestyle ever gets. I knew and understood the past, enjoyed the present, and had a good idea of what would happen in the future. Now I can claim no such confidence in any of those three verb tenses. I don't understand what happened in the past to put me at this point in the present, and I have no idea what the future has in store. All I know is that I am very far away from home, and I am absolutely terrified.

Chapter 12

Valentine's Day 2014
28°14'10.9"N 83°59'50.6"E
Pokhara, Nepal

Cassie and I show up at Quality Healthcare at 7:30 a.m. sharp. This time, I am not alone, and there should be no surprises. Today's blood sugar tests will confirm yesterday's, and I will be officially diagnosed with type 1 diabetes. Then, as soon as I can get on a flight, I am on my way home. And that is the only silver lining I can see in all this. This nightmare diagnosis in a foreign country, this change to everything I know and everything I knew, will be over soon, and I will begin to adjust my life to a new set of rules.

On our way over to the doctor's office, I keep thinking about one story that seems oddly appropriate. This is the one part in the story where my experience as a pilot is relevant.

On our first anniversary—the dating anniversary that only teens and newlyweds count, not the wedding anniversary—I rented a small four-seater plane and took Cassie to the Outer Banks of North Carolina. At the time, I was living in Norfolk, Virginia, so the flight to Ocracoke should've taken no more than ninety minutes. But an hour into the flight, as we passed Kitty Hawk, North Carolina, visibility suddenly dropped in what seemed like an opaque haze. I told Cassie we would spend the day in Kitty Hawk, not Ocracoke, and I turned the plane around.

I thought I was making a level turn, but as I looked down at my airspeed indicator, I realized I was at about 155 miles per hour— not an easy speed to obtain in an old-model Cessna 172. I must've

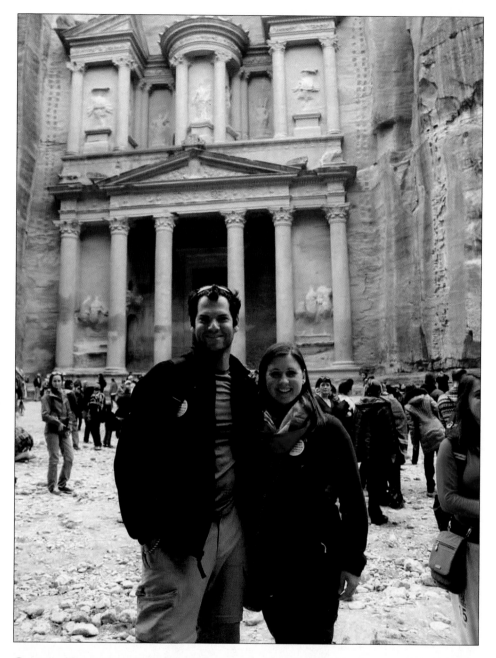

Cassie and I stand before the famous Treasury in Petra, Jordan. I had just started feeling the symptoms of diabetes, but I wouldn't know what they meant for nearly two more months.

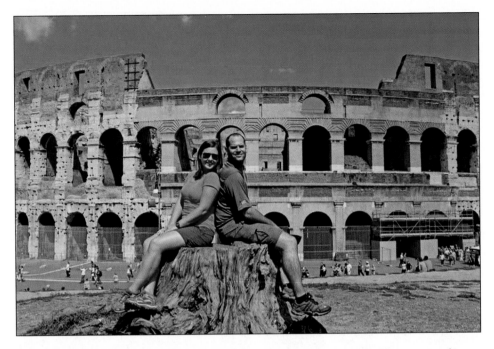

(Above) Cassie and I, posing in front of the Colosseum in Rome, Italy. This was our first picture together from the trip!

(Below) Guard post in Auschwitz-Birkenau in Poland.

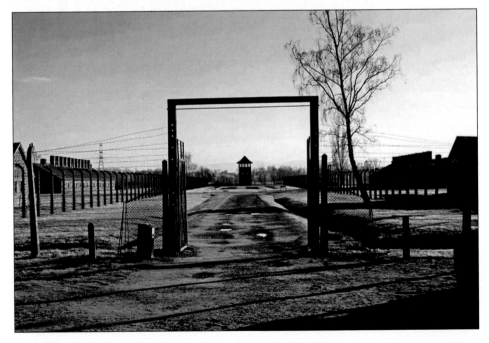

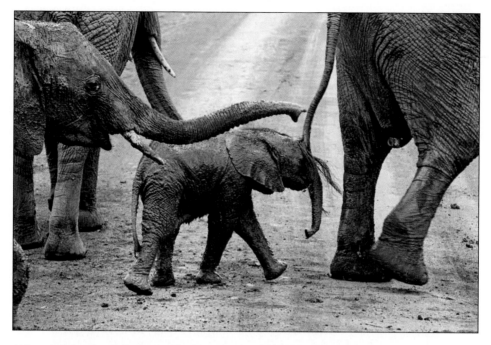

(Above) A family of elephants blocking the road in the Maasai Mara, Kenya. We were more than happy to admire them as they passed. Especially this little guy!

(Below) I have always been amazed by Cassie's ability to connect with children of different cultures. These kids speak only a few words of English, yet it didn't take long for them to learn how to give her a high five.

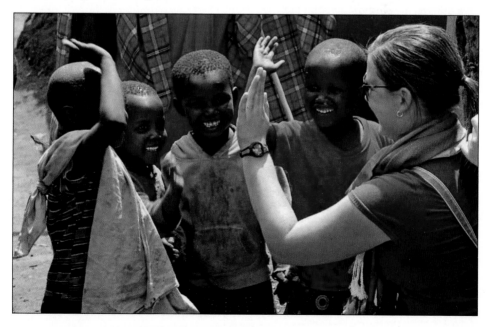

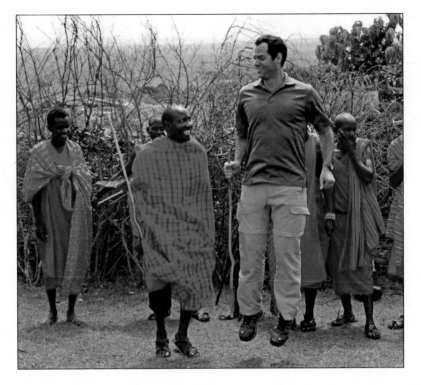

(Above) Maasai men measure their manhood by jumping. Despite my recently torn ACL, I think I earned their respect here.

(Below) The Songkan water festival in Laos meant constant splashing from all sides. Here, I am priming my weapon to return fire.

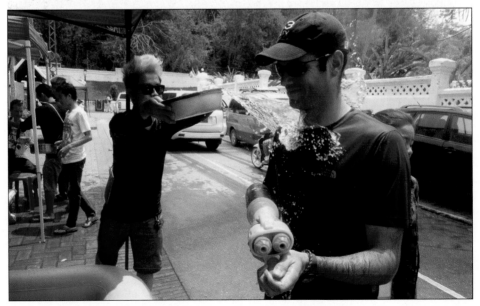

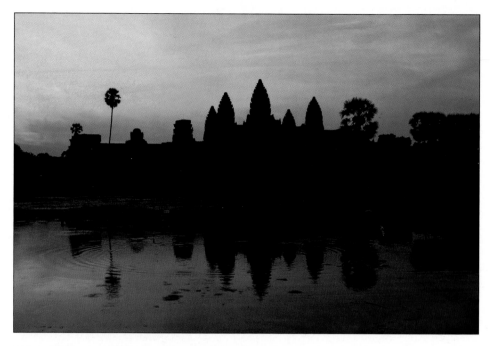

(Above) Sunrise over Angkor Wat in Cambodia. Worth every minute of standing by the mosquito-infested pool in front of us.

(Below) The temple of Bayon in Angkor, where hundreds of identical Buddha faces peer out from every corner.

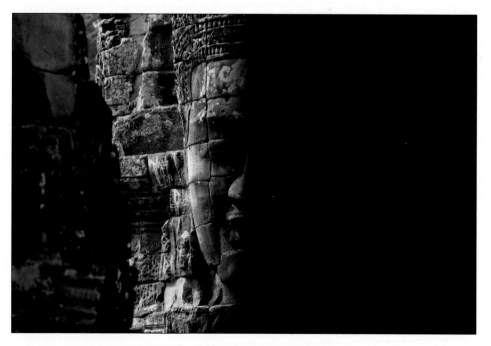

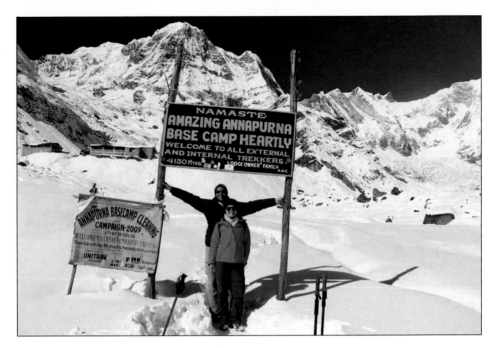

(Above) On our way down from Annapurna Base Camp in Nepal, after I had pushed my body past its breaking point.

(Below) Cassie in her natural element at Matepani Gumba in Nepal, teaching English to our young monks. I was the disciplinarian . . . and the photographer.

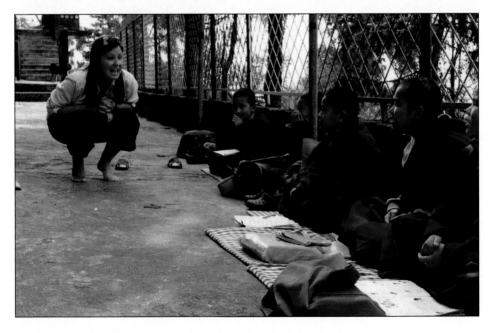

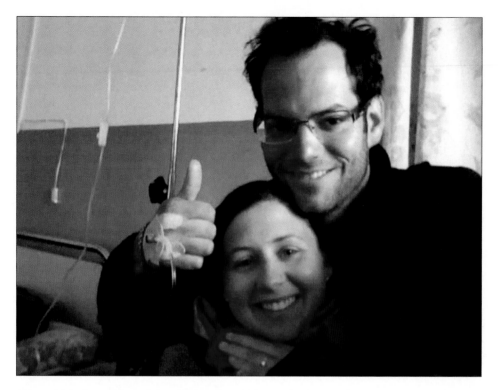

(Above) My first night at Dhital Educational Hospital in Nepal. I can still feel that IV in my hand.

(Below) Together with our Nepali hosts Bimala and Krishna—and the entire family.

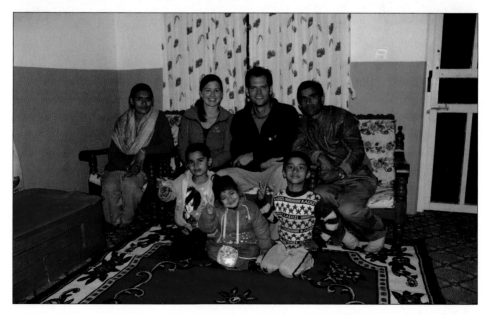

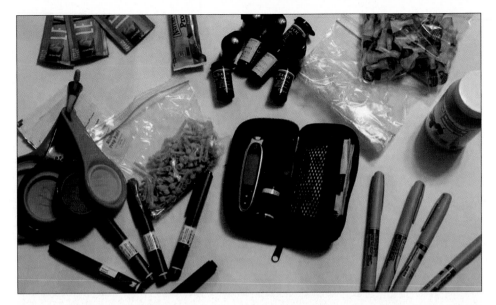

(Above) I packed my diabetic toolkit with everything I thought I would need. In this case, I was absolutely willing to overpack.

(Below) After my diagnosis, I wrote down every single one of my blood sugars, injections, and meals. It helped me get a better grip on diabetes quickly.

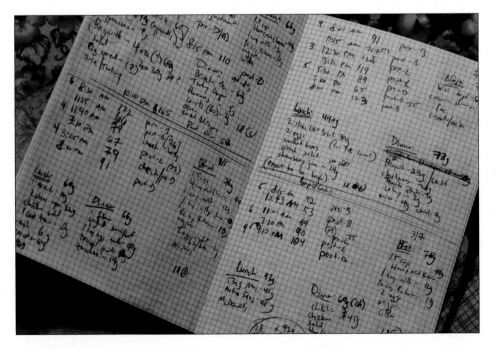

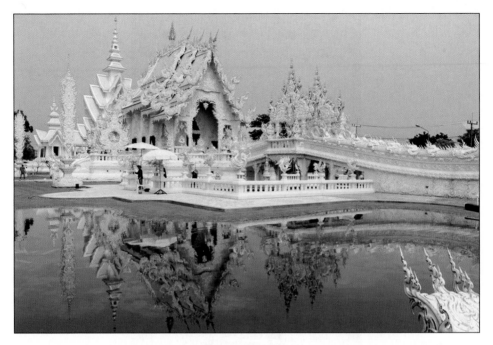

(Above) The White Temple in Chiang Rai, Thailand. It only gets weirder from here.

(Below) Throwing back a shot of cobra whiskey with a complete stranger in the Golden Triangle, Laos. Somehow, the fact that he was Canadian made me feel a bit better about our collective decision.

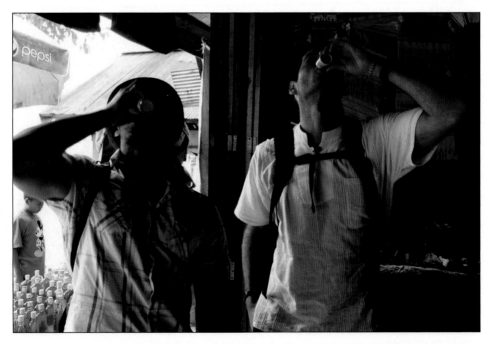

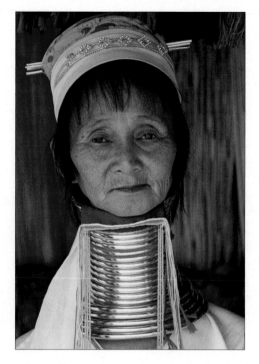

(Above) On our trip to Chiang Rai, we visited the Long Neck tribe. Exiles from Myanmar, they rely on tourists for their income.

(Below) An elephant statue in Wat Phanan Choeng temple in Ayutthaya, Thailand.

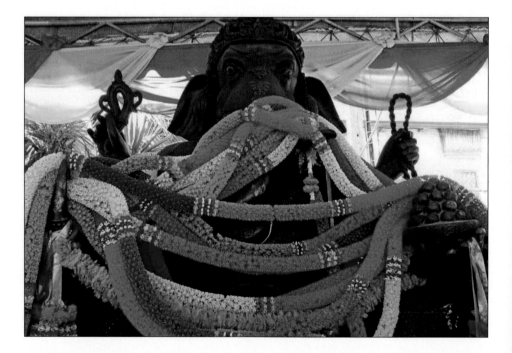

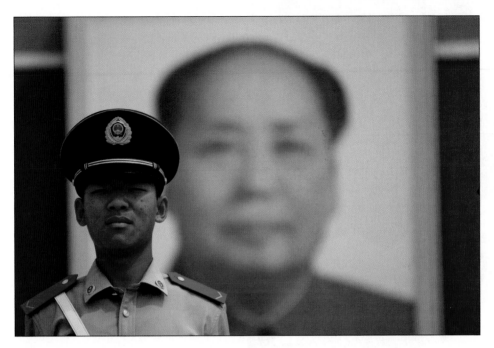

(Above) A Chinese soldier stands before a portrait of Mao Zedong. Beijing, China, is his world—we're just living in it.

(Below) Cassie hiking on a crumbling section along the Great Wall of China. This hike tested her fear of heights and my resolve to overcome the ravages of diabetes.

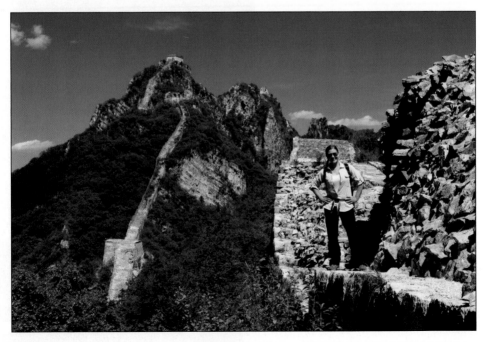

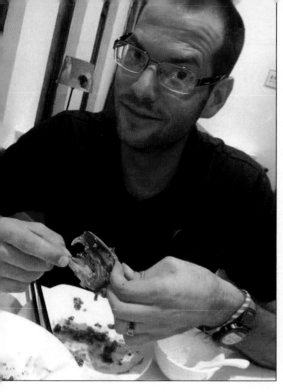

That moment you realize the rabbit leg you're eating in Beijing, China, has teeth and a jaw.

My parents traveled around Japan with us. Here, they pose in front of the gates of the Fushimi Inari Shrine in Kyoto, Japan.

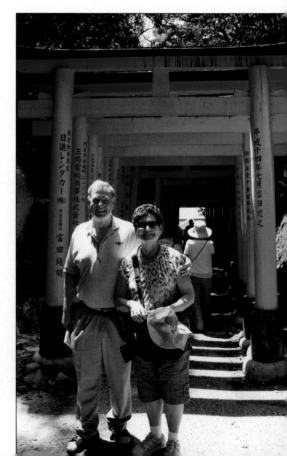

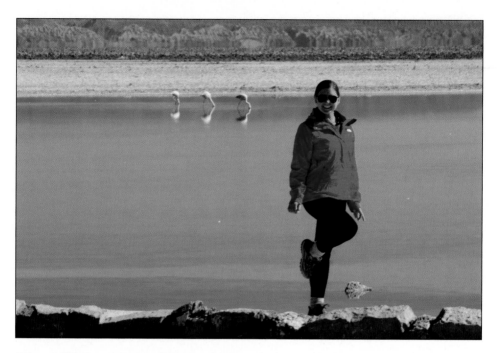

(Above) While visiting the Altiplanic Lagoons near San Pedro de Atacama in northern Chile, Cassie tried to act like the locals.

(Below) We bundled up against the bitter cold of the Altiplanic Lagoons, nestled into the seemingly extraterrestrial surface at 13,000 feet.

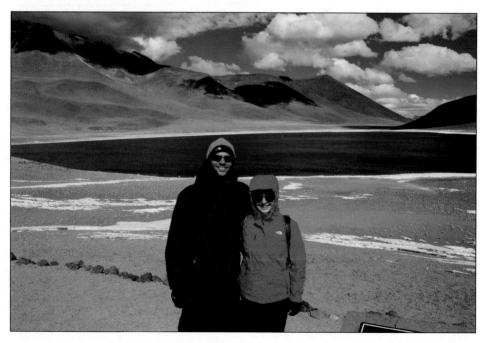

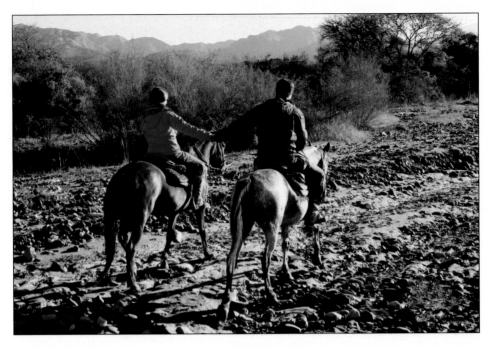

(Above) Given everything else we did on the trip, I shouldn't have been so excited to ride a horse in Salta, Argentina. And yet I enjoyed every moment atop my steed.

(Below) At the top of Dead Woman's Pass, Cassie and I pause for a photo before darkness sets in along the Inca Trail in Peru.

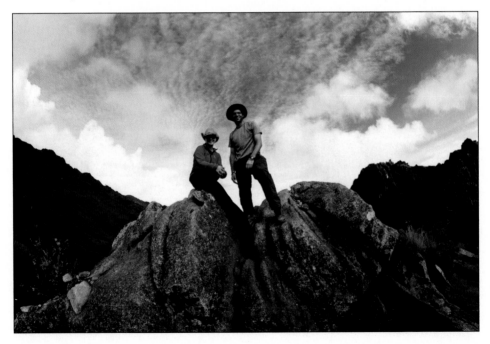

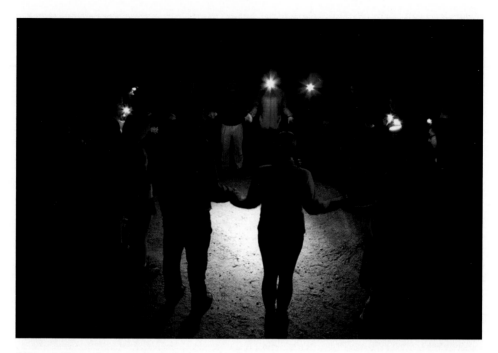

(Above) We woke up early in the morning for an intimate Incan meditation session before our final push to Machu Picchu.

(Below) What's the point of having diabetes if you can't have fun with it? I did my best Zen pose atop Huayna Picchu, 1,500 feet above Machu Picchu in Peru.

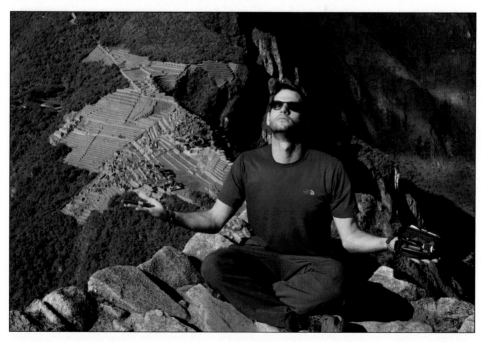

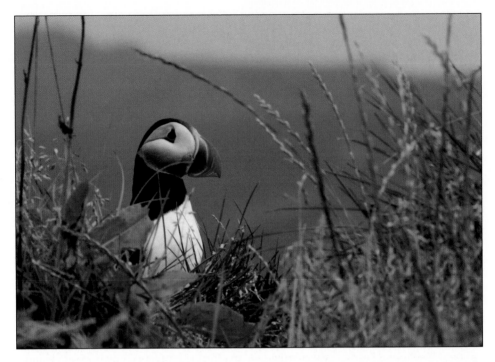

(Above) It's hard to believe the locals eat these colorful birds, but I wasn't heartless enough to try puffin meat in Reykjavik, Iceland. They're too cute!

(Below) Cassie and I pose for our last picture together from the trip on the water in Reykjavik. We are always looking forward to our next adventure.

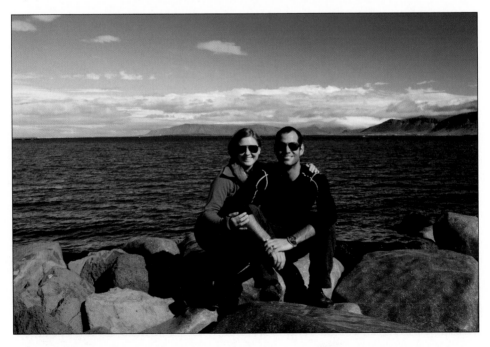

been descending, but when I checked outside the plane and glanced at the horizon, it didn't *look* like I was descending. Something was wrong, but I couldn't quite figure out what it was. Regardless, we landed at Kitty Hawk and spent the day hanging out at the beach.

In the early afternoon, the air filled with a thick, gray smoke. I'd covered enough fires as a journalist to know it wasn't house-fire smoke—it was wild-fire smoke, and it stank of the burning leaves and charred woods of a forest fire. As quickly as it came, it was gone, and the sky cleared. We enjoyed the rest of the afternoon on the beach, caught a movie when the sun got to be too much, then headed for the airport for the short flight home.

I checked the weather, and everything looked great. The possibility of thunderstorms—always a constant threat in the summer months—had passed with the afternoon heat, and we fired up the engine, looking for-ward to a beautiful flight home.

Only it turned out not to be so beautiful. Ten minutes into the flight, visibility again dropped to zero in thick haze. I was following Route 158, a road that goes straight from my origin to my destination, yet I found that I had to fly lower and lower to keep sight of the road. Before I knew it, I was down to 800 feet and still descending—dangerously low in a small airplane.

I kept flying north, hoping to break out of the clouds into clear weather. But it wasn't clouds. The more time we spent in the haze, the more I real-ized I was flying in smoke. The same smoke that had covered the beach a few hours earlier. And then it dawned on me. It was the same smoke that I'd flown into in the morning, only I hadn't been in it long enough to real-ize it was smoke. The worst wildfires in the country burned seventy miles away in North Carolina, and the winds pushed the smoke over the Outer Banks. As the wind shifted, the smoke drifted north, from Ocracoke, to Kitty Hawk, and now to Chesapeake, Virginia, where we were at that moment. Because smoke isn't a phenomenon of weather, it didn't show up in any meteorological charts that I checked.

I was in the worst kind of trouble. I hadn't yet finished my instrument rating—a certificate that lets me fly in zero visibility—and I was in a plane that wasn't well equipped for instrument flight. No GPS. No autopilot. And the weather was supposed to be so perfect that I hadn't brought my instru-ment charts. Young pilots in this situation survive an average of three min-utes, a statistic I decided not to tell Cassie.

Out of options and in need of immediate help, I hopped on the radio and called Norfolk air traffic control. It took about twenty minutes, but they got me lined up with Norfolk International Airport's runway and safely on the ground. Cassie and I had no problems polishing off a bottle of wine that night—not a standard bottle, but one of those big Yellow Tail bottles.

That night (before the wine), I talked to my flight instructor, and we broke down every moment of the flight and every decision I made, both good and bad. One thing he said always stuck with me.

He explained to me that experienced pilots with thousands of hours can sometimes get in trouble flying into zero visibility if they're not prepared for it. If they expect good weather and they get it, they're great. If they expect bad weather and get it, that's no problem. But if they expect good weather and find themselves flying in bad weather, they sometimes make very serious, very fatal, and very avoidable mistakes.

"Why? How is that possible?"

"Because the brain is wired for denial. Your brain wants you to believe that everything is going well. That everything is okay. Even when you face a growing list of things that are going wrong, your brain still wants you to think you're fine. The brain is wired for denial."

My instructor's final line keeps running through my mind as we make our way to the main road to catch a taxi to the doctor's office. The brain is wired for denial. Staying alive as a pilot is a matter of understanding and managing risk. Many of the lessons learned in the air can be applied to life. This is one of those lessons.

We arrive twenty minutes later for my fasting blood sugar test. A quick, cordial "hello" is exchanged, and Dr. Griffiths's assistant tests my blood sugar.

5 . . . 4 . . . 3 . . . 2 . . . 1 . . . 306.

My blood sugar is still sky high, and my diagnosis is confirmed. The third check after breakfast—my blood sugar is 319—is a formality to corroborate what we already know. I have type 1 diabetes. My official diagnosis comes on Valentine's Day. I ask the doctor for a urine test to check for ketones. I tell him I have a fruity taste in the back of my mouth. He conducts the test and, a short time later, says I have no ketones.

"You are okay to travel home," Dr. Griffiths reassures me in a way that is not at all reassuring.

Cassie and I race home. We have a busy afternoon before we catch our flight, and we have to work fast. But I am still feeling awful, and when we cross the gate to our host's house, I sit down on the stoop and cry.

"Are you okay?"

The brain is wired for denial.

I shake my head no.

"Do you want to go to the hospital now?"

The brain is wired for denial.

We have less than four hours until our flight to Kathmandu, where I know there is a modern hospital with doctors trained in Western schools, yet I feel too weak to last that long.

At some point, I had become addicted to the idea of my own health. I ignored all the warning signs, using excuses like being in a desert, hiking in the Himalayas, or being in Nepal during the dry season to explain my never-ending thirst and subsequent need to always run to the bathroom.

The notion of good health was a drug I could not do without, and as my health deteriorated, I kept increasing the dosage. My brain was wired for denial, and I had hardwired it to stay that way. I was unwilling to accept what would've been obvious to anyone else and perhaps even to myself if I weren't facing a constantly changing set of circumstances in an ever-growing list of locations.

I can do something about it now, or I can tell Cassie I don't want to go to the hospital, and I will be in Kathmandu at a Western clinic by dinnertime, only a few hours away. It would bring me one huge step closer to home, since it's much easier to coordinate a flight out of Kathmandu without the added complication of getting on one of the few daily flights from Pokhara to the capital.

But as much as I want to get home quickly—more than anything else in the world, I want to be with my parents in New Jersey—I feel too weak to last even a few more hours. The twenty-five-minute flight to Kathmandu feels like an eternity away, and if something goes wrong in the air, it's not like Nepal is littered with major airports we could divert to, let alone high-quality hospitals near those airports where I can find decent treatment.

It is time to play it safe, to break myself of the addiction to the fantasy of my own good health. I am in bad shape—very bad shape as I would learn—and I am getting worse. After misdiagnosing my symptoms, I come to believe the doctor in Pokhara misdiagnosed the severity of my condition.

So when Cassie asks, "Do you want to go to the hospital?" the answer is . . .

"Yes."

A moment later, we tell the cab driver to bring us to Dhital Educational Hospital. The first stage of my journey home had been so close. A few hours away, it was an imminent reality. Now, it is once again a distant dream. There may be some sort of light at the end of a proverbial tunnel, but the tunnel keeps getting longer and the light in the distance is fading.

We walk straight into the emergency room of what looks like a large, modern medical center. Inside the emergency room, blood stains the floor, along with other bodily fluids that I'd rather not attempt to identify. There is no heater here, so even though the daytime temperature is quite warm, it's freezing inside the hospital. In the bed next to me is a young girl who keeps vomiting on herself, her bed, and the floor. The least repugnant and most pleasant object in the room to stare at is the ceiling, so I keep my concentration focused straight up as I wait for medical attention.

The doctors run every conceivable test on me over the next two hours. Blood tests, urine tests, ultrasounds, x-rays, even an HIV test. I find out I have a six-millimeter kidney stone, which the technician describes as "small, do not worry," but to me sounds absolutely enormous. At every test, I am pushed to the front of the line. This is racism in reverse. As all the Nepalis wait their turn, I am tested immediately because the hospital knows I have money. The battery of tests costs a total of four thousand Nepali rupees—forty dollars.

I am brought to the room in the special ward of the hospital that will be my world until I am discharged. As we come to learn, "special" means "foreigner." The Nepalis stay in the general ward, which is a fancy term for what is actually the lobby. They simply lie down on a mat around the nurses' desk and sleep on the floor every night until they are discharged. The setup resembles camping far more than it does emergency medical care. About twenty or thirty Nepalis are in the general ward when I walk through. I can't imagine what this ward must look like when the hospital is busy.

My room is the last room at the end of the hall on the left. When I arrive, I am the only person in the special ward. This room is far too expensive for your average Nepali—it costs ten dollars a night—so the hospital reserves this ward for Westerners who suffer altitude sickness on a trek or catch a stomach bug in town. I wonder if I'm the first Westerner to be admitted with newly diagnosed diabetes.

We have two beds. I take the one by the window; Cassie takes the bed by the door. The hospital has no Wi-Fi, so Cassie has to run out to email my parents that I'm in the hospital. And since our room is freezing cold, she goes to pick up our sleeping bags. They got us through a Himalayas trek; they'll get us through a few nights in a hospital.

A nurse immediately sticks an IV on the back of my right hand, between my middle and ring fingers, and starts pumping fluids into me. In my first forty-eight hours in the hospital, I gain about fifteen pounds. That's how dehydrated I was. My body was missing two gallons of water, which explains why I was constantly thirsty and why my skin looked like it was hanging off my face and arms those last few days.

We see the first doctor fairly quickly. He is middle-aged, maybe in his early forties, dressed fairly casually, as if my admittance to the hospital disrupted his other plans for the day. He doesn't smile or betray any emotion but speaks to me very matter-of-factly in a monotone he must've learned in one of his med school electives. This doctor isn't Nepali; he's Indian, and so are all of the other doctors here. He is accompanied by a team of med students, all wearing lab coats, and they are using me as a lesson. For my entire stay in the hospital, every time I see a doctor, med students follow him—here the doctor is always a *him*—plucking up kernels of advice that fall from the mother hen.

He explains my situation and treatment to me, including how soon I'll be given my first shot of insulin, but there is only one question that interests me.

"Our goal is to get home as quickly as possible. How long will I be in the hospital?"

"We need to flush the ketones and maybe twenty-four hours after that. So maybe two days."

For the first time in a long time, I feel optimistic. This stretch of feeling weak and awful has an end in sight, and I will be on my way home soon.

"What do I eat?"

"Oh, do not worry. We have a diabetic menu we will bring you."

"Thank you, Doctor. Thank you very much."

Then a nurse arrives and hands Cassie a list of supplies to buy, and we realize we are very, very far from Western medical care. We assumed this hospital would work like any hospital in the States. We get treated, they give us a bill, we go home. If we stay long enough, they give us the right food. It's a simple arrangement that I didn't think needed improvement.

In Nepal, it's almost the exact opposite. You pay for everything up front, including supplies, medicines, and tests. Then you bring it to the nurse, and the nurse administers the medicines. Cassie is sent on a scavenger hunt throughout the hospital complex to find the medical supplies store, the pharmacy, and the payment window, none of which are located near each other. Then, after she finishes those errands, she has to go to the cafeteria to buy me food, since it's not served to patients here. The food consists of the same vegetable curry and rice that we've eaten since arriving in Nepal, only now it's served in little plastic bags instead of on plates. They're reluctant to give Cassie a tray with my food since they fear she may not return it after I finish eating.

I never quite figured out how I would've gotten all the supplies and my meals without Cassie. Did they really expect me to walk around the entire hospital to get everything I need? Forget the fact that I'm incredibly weak for a second. I'm hooked up to an IV, and they don't have the IV stands on wheels like they do in the States. My IV hangs from an immovable pole attached to my bed. For me to walk around, I need to unhook my IV bag, hold it high in my left hand, and keep my right hand down so the fluid keeps going. Is that what would've happened? God, I hope not, but that's exactly what I have to do every time I go to the bathroom, holding my IV bag above my head in my left hand and my penis in my right hand. If I were to try it the other way round, blood would flow out of my hand into the IV bag.

The doctor returns to my hospital room after a few hours. "I would like you to move to the intensive care unit. We can monitor you better there." The doctor gives us his pitch as to why I should switch from my luxurious corner office to the ICU. "You can take a look at the intensive care unit. It is across from the nurses' station."

Cassie and I walk down together. We are shocked by what we see. Or rather, who we see. A dozen beds are lined up against the walls, spaced five or six feet apart. I think each bed is occupied, but I don't stick around long enough to double-check. That's because everyone in the ICU looks like they're about to die. Each patient is hooked up to an aging array of medical devices, yet the beeps and bings of the medical machinery don't seem to be helping. Every patient looks like they are moments away from passing on. If I wait long enough, they may be able to relabel this room "The Morgue." I have no doubt that I would receive better care here (and they have heat in this room!), but I refuse to let the hospital treat me like my life is in imminent danger of ending. As politely as we can, we tell the doctor there is no fucking way I'm switching to the intensive care unit. Thankfully, he doesn't argue. He just asks me to sign a waiver releasing the hospital from any liability.

The first night in the hospital is the only night that qualifies as not bad. We have a room with a TV, so we watch whatever Olympic sport is coming in on the sports channels. I catch up on curling, downhill skiing, and a random assortment of other winter events. The nurses wake me up every two hours to take my vitals, which means I barely sleep, but I don't mind too much. I am on the mend, and that means more to me than a few hours of rest. I sleep with most of my body enclosed in the warmth of my mummy bag; only my right arm is outside so I don't risk unhooking my IV.

I wish I could say the emotional breakdowns stop, but they don't. Everything that's happened is still nearly impossible for me to comprehend. Just a few months ago, I was perfectly healthy, wandering around Europe without a care in the world. Now I'm in a hospital in Pokhara, Nepal, trying to figure out how close I came to killing myself with undiagnosed type 1 diabetes on a trek through the Himalayas.

When we wake up, Cassie and I work out a simple system to make sure I'm okay while keeping my family informed. She will sleep in Lakeside and spend the whole day with me in the hospital. That way, she can send emails and check in with my family at night and in the morning since the hospital has no way of accessing the Internet. Apparently, the term *World Wide Web* does not apply to the entire world, but it has an alliterative feel that, I must admit, is far more appealing than *Partial Wide Web*.

On our first full day in the hospital, I tell Cassie it's okay to post my diagnosis on Facebook. Only one or two of my friends know I have diabetes, and that seems the most efficient way to let everyone know.

I am not ready for what comes next. Cassie walks in each morning with a new stack of messages from friends and strangers, each and every one offering their love and support. People I haven't spoken with in years send short notes that become so powerful for me. Even something as simple as "Thinking of you, Oren! Feel better soon," or "I just learned of what is going on. I love you and know you will end up adjusting to all of this," makes each minute in the hospital just a little bit easier. I find it difficult to read more than a few messages at a time without crying. I've never experienced such an outpouring of unfiltered emotional support, and there is no way to hold back my own emotions as I go through the messages.

After Josh had his stroke, I saw him cry as he read the messages of support he received. It didn't quite make sense to me then. I thought they would make him smile. At the time, I told him to man up. Grow some balls. Quit your bitching. This is good advice, and I'm sticking with it. But I get it now. I understand why these messages can be so emotional. More important, I understand how critical they are in the healing process. While the body recovers, so, too, must the soul. And just as Jen was so important to Josh when he was in the hospital, Cassie is that important to me, if not more so.

We settle into our own little routine for a couple of days. Neither of us is particularly worried about my health at this point. I have diabetes, and I am in a hospital. Certainly I'm no expert, but I'm pretty sure no one has died of newly diagnosed diabetes while still at the hospital. Yet on the other side of the Atlantic, mass hysteria has sprouted roots in the Liebermann household.

My parents want by-the-minute updates that are simply impossible to give. The hospital barely gives me any information about my own health, and without Wi-Fi or a calling card, I have no way of imparting this knowledge with anything resembling alacrity to my parents halfway around the world. We quickly realize that the only thing that happens quickly here is us realizing that nothing happens quickly here. They draw blood each morning to test my blood sugar, but I don't learn the results until late in the afternoon, which is like a nurse taking your temperature at breakfast but not finding out what the thermometer said until dinner. Same thing for a ketone test. They ask for a urine sample the second they walk in every morning, but I don't find out anything about my ketone levels for another eight hours.

The difference in time zones works against us. My parents want a constant stream of information. They want to know what's going on right before they go to bed, and they want an email waiting in their inbox right when they wake up. But since we're eleven hours and forty-five minutes ahead of Eastern Standard Time—a difference they fail to take into account—their eight hours of sleep is right in the middle of our day when there are absolutely no worthwhile updates. And our eight hours of sleep are in the middle of their day, when they fanatically check their inboxes for our messages. At first, their emails come every few hours. "How are you feeling? What is your latest blood sugar? What are the doctors telling you?" Soon, they start coming every few minutes, to the point where we wake up in the morning with a chronological firing squad of frantic messages, each a little more panicked than the last.

It is the worry and concern of loving parents manifested in the growing fear of distant ignorance. They are afraid because they don't know enough not to be afraid, and they can't do anything about it because they're halfway around the world. I become convinced that my mom thinks I have late-stage bubonic plague, not type 1 diabetes. I tell them not to buy flight tickets to Nepal, since I plan on being out of the hospital by the time they would arrive.

In the isolation of a disconnected hospital, I am insulated from their never-ending stream of emails and messages. Instead, Cassie bears the full force of the digital onslaught. She has a raw deal: she has to take care of me in the hospital and my parents at home. For the only time all week, the tears come from *her* eyes and not mine.

"I just don't know how much longer I can do this. I can't be here with you and responding to all of their emails."

"I'll write an email to my folks. Send it to them when you get Wi-Fi."

My words have no effect, and the frantic messages continue at the same unabated pace as before, leaving Cassie in a miserable situation.

The doubts about the quality of medical care I'm receiving creep their way into my mind on the third day in the hospital. I should be leaving today. All of the doctors predicted I would be on my way home by now, but we keep hearing the same answer every time we ask about leaving.

"We need to stabilize your blood sugar levels and flush the ketones. That will take another twenty-four to forty-eight hours. Then we will be ready to discharge you." The doctors say it as if they're reading off a cue card. It's the same thing we've been hearing for three straight days.

Meanwhile, every doctor back in the States has said I shouldn't be in the hospital more than two or three days. It doesn't take that long to regulate blood sugar and clear the system of ketones. On top of that, I still haven't gotten the diabetic menu I'm supposed to be eating, so Cassie and I guess at what I should be eating and how much of it to eat. We are very much the blind leading the blind.

My blood sugars are still in the mid to high 200s, and I feel helpless. Even Cassie, who has done her best to radiate eternal optimism, is wearing down. I want to go home, and yet that seems no more plausible now than it did when I arrived at the hospital. For the first and only time during our stay in Pokhara, the sky is covered in a thick layer of solid overcast. Normally this sort of weather clears very quickly here, but now it is here for days. The darkness seeps through the window and into the hospital and into my room, draining me of any positive energy. The frigid temperatures have worked their way into my very core. I shiver at night in my sleeping bag, waiting and hoping and praying for all of this to end.

The third night in the hospital is the hardest and longest night of my life.

When Cassie leaves for the evening to update friends and family, I am left alone with my thoughts and a TV that has a bewildering array of random channels, all of which are categorically unable to distract me from my present condition. There is no clock in the room, so I have no way of judging time. Seconds and minutes tick away in a relentless grind that I cannot measure.

In a week of hardship, these are my worst moments.

These are my darkest hours.

I try to stay awake as long as I can, watching whatever sport I can find—I watch more cricket during my time in the hospital than I've ever watched before—hoping that when I open my eyes again, Cassie will be there. If I fall asleep too early, I'll have to wake up and wait for her arrival in the morning, and I don't know if I can handle that. I want to face the morning and a new day knowing she is by my side.

The movie *Contraband* comes on a random channel around midnight, and I stay up watching the entire flick, happy to have something in English to watch that doesn't require me to learn the rules of an entirely new and apparently nonsensical sport. It's certainly not Mark Wahlberg's greatest film, but it gives me something on which to focus my thoughts for its full 109 minutes, and for that, I am eternally grateful.

"How's it going, babe?" Cassie asks when she arrives on my fourth day at the hospital. "How was last night?"

"It's tough. I just want to go home. I feel like I'm going to be here forever." I take a deep breath. "And I can't get any goddamn answers around here," I whisper. After carefully discussing and considering all of our options, the pros and cons, risks and rewards, and costs and benefits, we make a very serious decision.

In short, fuck this place. We're leaving tomorrow. Mark, the missionary doctor in Kathmandu we happen to know through Cassie's church, recommends a Western clinic there, and he promises good care and warm beds, two things that seem to be in very short supply at this hospital that has become my prison these last few days.

We expect a fight in the morning when we tell the doctors about our plans to leave. Instead, they tell me that I'm well enough to go and that I'm barely producing any ketones anymore. They tell me I'm healthy. My bullshit alarm goes off, but I keep quiet as we discuss my time in the hospital.

"Have you been eating the food we recommend for diabetics?"

"No. I never got the diabetic menu."

"Okay, we will make sure that you get that immediately."

"Doctor, don't I need some way of testing my blood sugar on the way home?"

"No, you do not need to test your blood sugar. You will be fine," he says in a way that somehow introduces more doubt than comfort.

An hour later, I still haven't received any inkling of a hint about a diabetic menu. I go ballistic. I'm no longer hooked up to the IV—I get two bottles of fluids a day, but I'm not constantly connected like I was during my first two days here—so I storm down the hallway and toward the nurses' desk wearing my black CBS fleece atop my gray T-shirt. That part of me looks somewhat normal. But I'm wearing athletic shorts and wool socks pulled up over my calves. That part of me looks insane. I verbally assault the first nurse that looks my way.

"I was told I'd have a diabetic menu three days ago. Then I was told I'd have one an hour ago, and I'm still waiting. I want to know what's taking so long." This is not a country accustomed to raised voices and pointing fingers. My words have the effect of a torrent of curses, even without interlacing my language with the liberal application of colorful profanity.

"I'm sorry, we will have someone bring it to you as soon as possible."

Out of the corner of my eye, I spot the menu. It's been sitting here on the nurses' desk—for how long I have no idea—and I realize immediately why it wasn't brought to me. No one finished translating it. The breakfast menu and part of the lunch menu are in English, but the rest is missing. A piece of paper that's clearly the Nepali menu sits right below it.

"Is that my menu? Why haven't you finished translating it? I want someone to translate it right now, while I'm waiting here!"

A nurse grabs the pieces of paper, takes one look at them, and then puts them aside. For the first time in my life, I am tempted to deliver a flying uppercut to a medical professional, perhaps with an emphatic *hadoken* or *shoryuken*.

"You know what? Just give me that."

"You speak Nepali?" This is the nurse's attempt at humor at my expense.

"No, but I can learn faster than you can translate." In all honesty, I didn't say that—I should have—but one of the residents comes over at that moment and finishes translating the menu. My effort is nonetheless pointless. The doctors have already agreed to let me leave early the next morning. I don't care about anything else at the moment. I just don't want to be here anymore.

I barely sleep my fourth and final night at Dhital Educational Hospital. I'm too excited. In my four days at the hospital, I have left my room only twice. Now I am leaving for good. When Cassie shows up in the morning, we quickly grab our belongings, sign out of the hospital—we have to wait for them to hand copy my medical notes since apparently they have no copier—and head for the hotel room that has been Cassie's home while I have been infirm. She throws her stuff together while I hop in the shower. I didn't bother showering at the hospital because they didn't have hot water. That wouldn't have been a problem if the room had any semblance of heat, but there was no fucking way I was taking a freezing cold shower in a freezing cold room. Diabetes is enough to deal with. I'd rather not have to fend off pneumonia as well.

We race over to Krishna and Bimala's house to say goodbye to our host family one final time. I haven't seen Bimala or the kids since I went to the hospital—Krishna stopped by to check up on me—and I embrace them all like the family they have become. It may be years before I see them again, but I have no doubt this is not our last time together.

Then it's off to the airport for the short flight to Kathmandu. We haven't had our bags fully packed since we arrived in Nepal six weeks ago. I couldn't have imagined then what I'd be going through now, but this is my reality.

On the twenty-five-minute flight, I keep hoping the doctors at the Western clinic will clear me to fly home immediately. Then we don't have to unpack. We can head straight back to the airport and buy tickets for the next flight out. No more nights of waiting. No more horrible uncertainty about the immediate future. I can just go home.

We called ahead from Pokhara, so the staff at the clinic, called CIWEC, is expecting us. A nurse leads me into an examination room and immediately puts an IV in my left hand, just below the wrist. She draws blood to test my blood sugar.

When the doctor sees me a short time later, I tell him my diagnosis and my experience at the last hospital. He looks over my medical notes for a moment.

"I think you should stay here for at least two days. We need to regulate your blood sugars and teach you to use insulin before we can let you fly home." My dreams of catching a flight home tonight have vanished. Worse than that, the doctor's treatment plan sounds exactly like the plan from the last hospital.

The nurse returns with the results of my blood test. My blood sugar is 320, and my ketones are 3+, the highest reading on the scale. Ketones are a byproduct of dangerously high blood sugars and happen when there is not enough insulin in the system. The condition that arises is called diabetic ketoacidosis, where the body poisons itself. Untreated, it can be fatal, and before the invention of artificial insulin, it nearly always was. Theoretically, it should be easy to treat with modern medicine, but I had spent five days at a hospital that's considered the best in Pokhara, and for all of the doctors I saw and all of the tests they ran, they managed to do absolutely nothing except hydrate me. My blood sugar is still through the roof, and my body is still poisoning itself.

Once again, I feel like I'm going nowhere. We took one huge step toward home by moving from Pokhara to Kathmandu—we are now a short cab ride away from the only place we can catch a flight home—but that still feels like an eternity away. Cassie and I bring our bags up to our room on the second floor. I wonder how long we'll be here, and if this room will turn into the same prison cell that the last room became.

Dr. Kishore Pandey comes into the room after we settle in. He is the doctor that advised us to stay at least two days, so he's already fairly high on my shit list at the moment. But he's smiling, and that automatically scores him a few redemption points. As he describes to me what will happen over the next few days, he is straightforward and honest, looking me right in the eye, yet he speaks with a warmth and empathy that melt away any frustration I had at being stuck in Nepal even longer. For the first time in two weeks, I am in front of a doctor who makes me believe he knows what he's talking about—a not inconsiderable feat considering how many doctors I've seen—and I realize I am in a far better place with infinitely better medical care. And—thank Moses—my room has heat. The staff at CIWEC is even happy to move the Wi-Fi router so we have a good signal in our room.

Dr. Pandey throws away the plan from the old hospital. He takes me off the insulin they gave me and switches me to two different types of insulin. He sits with us for maybe forty-five minutes, explaining diabetes and its short- and long-term complications, as he teaches me not only how to regulate blood sugar but what it means to have blood sugar readings that are too high or too low. We learn more in five minutes with him than we did in five days at Dhital Educational Hospital.

"Our endocrinologist will be in tomorrow morning to see you. If you need me, I will be right across the hall," he says after we finish with my first lesson in diabetes management. Cassie and I busy ourselves emailing my family to fill them in on the flight to Kathmandu and the new hospital. We give my parents my phone number, and they check in twice a day.

Sleep comes much easier on this night. Cassie has her own bed in the room, and we both know I'm in a better place. I allow myself to be a bit hopeful that we will be home soon. It is a dangerous hope, one that I have had too often this past week, and that dream has turned out to be untrue so many times. Now, maybe it will finally happen.

The moment I wake up, I go through the regular routine of blood tests and vital signs that has become nearly metronomic at this point. Dr. Jyoti Bhattarai sees me in the morning, and just like Dr. Pandey before her, she knows how to put a patient at ease and convey the impression that, with her care, you will get better, not worse. She reviews a lot of what Dr. Pandey talked about, then looks over my notes. She creates an entirely new insulin regimen for me, and she says she'll be back tomorrow to check my numbers and make any necessary adjustments to my new plan.

"Do you have any questions?"

"Just one, Doctor. We want to go home as soon as possible. When do you think we'll be able to leave?"

I hold my breath. I've asked this question of every doctor we've seen and haven't gotten a real answer yet.

"I think you will be healthy enough to fly home tomorrow afternoon."

I could jump up and hug her for that answer. There is no hesitation or doubt in her voice. Unless something goes wrong, she says she'll be more than happy to discharge me tomorrow.

Cassie and I order lunch from the restaurant next door—standard practice at this hospital—elated at the good news. I don't even mind when the nurses come in to teach Cassie how to administer insulin. They take turns pinching small bundles of fat on my stomach and sticking me with the short needles. Now I know what it's like to be a human test subject, and if I had any tears to spare, I would have shed one for all the rats that unwittingly devote themselves to medical experimentation.

We check flight schedules and find a flight on Etihad Airways that leaves late tomorrow night. Cassie calls the airline's Kathmandu office and asks them to hold two tickets. Dr. Bhattarai will check in with us this afternoon by phone and give us the go ahead to make the purchase.

Two hours after lunch, I'm sending an email to my parents, giving them the medical update and mentally preparing myself for a long journey home. It is time to test my blood sugar with my small hoard of newly acquired diabetes supplies. Instead of waiting eight hours for the results, I have only to wait a few seconds. It is, I notice, the same type of blood sugar monitor from a week ago when I was first diagnosed. The numbers tick down.

5 . . . 4 . . . 3 . . . 2 . . . 1 . . . 152.

It is 1:50 p.m. local time on my sixth day at the hospital—February 19, 2014—and though this time and date have absolutely no significance to the vast majority of people out there, they are so important to me that I write them down, never to forget this exact moment. Ever since I started showing symptoms of diabetes eight weeks ago, my blood sugar had been sky high. Even after getting medical help a week ago, my blood sugar was still too high. Finally, after five days spent in two different hospitals, my blood sugar is normal. Well, almost normal, but I couldn't care less about *almost* in this situation.

For the first time all week, the tears I shed are tears of joy. I am going home. I will hug my family and laugh with my friends and learn about my disease, and I will do that all from the comfort of my parents' house. When we speak with Dr. Bhattarai on the phone, she is thrilled for me, and she says it's fine for us to buy tickets.

Cassie races over to the Etihad Airways office and purchases two business class seats on Flight 293 from Kathmandu to Abu Dhabi and on Flight 101 from Abu Dhabi to JFK. It is the only time on our trip we are not sitting in economy, a welcome respite from our shoestring budget. My parents told us they would pay for the seats to make sure that, if I needed any help or medical attention, I would get it immediately. My sister's husband, Cam, who is on a business trip in Dubai, will meet us at the airport and hang out with us during our ten-hour layover. Then my parents will meet us at JFK when we step foot on American soil once again.

I email my family, expecting their responses of "Safe travels!" and "See you soon!" to clog up all available bandwidth in Nepal. Instead, we get crickets. Not a single response for hours. My entire family was all too happy to send a thousand emails for every small bit of bad news, but now that I'm finally coming home, everyone has apparently lost interest.

The rest of the time in the hospital flies by. One more night and one more day. Dr. Bhattarai stops in to see me one more time before our flight. She makes a small adjustment to my insulin regimen, and wishes us a safe trip home. Cassie snaps a picture of me standing with Dr. Bhattarai and Dr. Pandey. I have known these two doctors for only two days, yet I will be eternally grateful for the help they have given me. I give them each a big hug. I don't particularly care if I violate any of Nepal's social norms by hugging people I barely know, but it's the only way I know to express my gratitude.

We stay at the hospital until it's time to head for the airport. I'm getting antsy, ready for us to be on our way, and I can sense Cassie feels the same way.

"Do you think you'll want to finish our trip?" she asks.

"Yes, absolutely."

"How long do you want to be home for?"

"I don't know. Maybe four to six weeks? Does that sound okay?"

"Yeah, I was thinking the same thing."

An email pops up in my inbox. I see it's from my mom, so I open it up.

Wed, Feb 19, 2014 at 10:11 p.m.
Yaffa Liebermann
To: Liebermann Family

Subject: Cotton Candy

Hi my children

Cotton candy is my favorite from childhood.

Just for the fun of it I am sharing this picture. We went to the famous restaurant: "farmajrry" in Random (my mom's typing trails off here).

It it still a nice evening.

Love you.

I can't believe what I've just read. Less than a week after I'm diagnosed with type 1 diabetes, my mom sends out an email about how much she loves cotton candy, including a picture with a giant wad of pink, fluffy sugar. She is smiling and ripping off a piece with her right hand. I read it to Cassie, and we start laughing. My mom has just sent what might be the most colossally insensitive email in the history of the digital age. I've never once seen her eat cotton candy, and the only time she does it is shortly after I've gotten the news that cotton candy can now kill me.

At 5:00 p.m., we catch a cab to the airport and board our first flight. The five-hour hop puts us in Abu Dhabi at midnight. Cam is waiting for us as we exit the airport. He stayed mostly quiet during the countless family email exchanges of the past week. He knew if I needed his help, I would reach out for it, and I knew he would be there for me if I needed him. I saw him only two months ago in Kenya, but so much has changed in the intervening period. In many ways, I am a very different person than I was then.

I bum-rush Cam as he's standing there peacefully. He is not ready for the force I exert upon his chest and back when I give him a hug. He is the first member of my family I've seen since my diagnosis, and it feels absolutely exhilarating.

We drive around Abu Dhabi for an hour, seeing some of the city's highlights at night while we chat about everything that's happened. In the morning, we head for the airport once more, this time for the flight home.

The flight itself is almost completely uneventful. Cassie shoots me up with insulin before meals, partially because the nurses taught her how to do it, but also because my eyesight goes in and out of focus constantly. I don't know why it's happening, but I don't care at the moment. I'll figure that out on American soil. A few hours from home, I pull up the map of our flight on my TV screen.

"That's odd," I think. It shows us heading to Washington, DC, not New York. Once again, I'm not concerned. I figure someone must've configured the map incorrectly, until the captain comes over the intercom and explains what's happening. Flights into JFK are backed up because of weather. We're diverting to Dulles until the delays are sorted out.

Will this fucking journey home never end! We spend four hours on the tarmac at Dulles—thankfully, I'm tired enough that I sleep most of the time—before we are finally able to fly to our original destination. We have no way of knowing it yet, but this will become a common theme on our trip. Every time we try to return to American soil, something always goes wrong.

We touch down at JFK late in the evening. I hand Cassie the camera to snap a photo of the moment I hug my parents. My dad is first. He is standing right outside of the international arrivals door, and we spot each other instantly.

The ensuing embrace is a bear hug of epic proportions. We both refuse to let go. I'm not sure if he's happier to see me or the other way around. Either way, we are thrilled to be together again.

This place seemed so far away a few short days ago, but for everything I don't know—about my health, about our future, about our plans—one thing is certain.

I am home.

Chapter 13

February 25, 2014
40°19'14.6"N 74°04'23.4"W
Shrewsbury, New Jersey

I have never particularly enjoyed any visit to a medical professional, and my recent medical interactions have only reinforced my already negative predisposition. Since the odds are high that I will be poked, prodded, injected, tested, and examined, I find the entire experience rather unpleasant, especially if that medical professional happens to be a dentist. There is no earthly moral justification for one human being to insert electric drills, sharp picks, or pliers into the mouth of another human being, and, yes, I did once have a dentist pull out a tooth with pliers, an experience that was so awful that it haunts me to this very day.

Another dentist even said to me, "You have very nice teeth, and you need a root canal." These two thoughts cannot possibly go together. In point of fact, they are diametrically opposed.

That being said, I will make an exception on this day. And only on this day.

Once I booked my tickets home from Nepal, my parents immediately scheduled a doctor's appointment for me with our family physician. I haven't seen him in years, not since I was right out of college, but within a few minutes of sitting with him on my first Tuesday back home, I remember why my parents trust him so much. Dr. Robert Carracino doesn't have any superpowers as a healer, and he isn't exceptional in some diagnostic field. He even looks fairly normal— a middle-aged man with dark hair who keeps himself in very good shape by cycling regularly. But he has far more valuable skills. He is honest, knowledgeable, and straightforward.

"How did I suddenly get diabetes?" I ask him.

"There's no way to tell. It could be a virus you picked up somewhere. You could have been sick for half a day. And that's it. The virus plants itself in your pancreas, and when your body goes to shut down the virus, it shuts down the pancreas."

If you're looking for a more thorough explanation as to how I developed juvenile diabetes at thirty-one years of age or what biological processes were happening inside my body, you've come to the wrong place, partly because I know little of medicine, but mostly because medicine knows little of type 1 diabetes. Answers to those questions don't exist yet, at least not with any degree of certainty, and they may not exist for a long time. Doctors and scientists still have no idea what causes a pancreas to fail so spectacularly and unexpectedly, and my hapless pancreas is no exception.

I was sick for two days right when Cassie and I got to Israel, and that's when the thirst began. As I see it, that's the most likely starting point for my diabetes. Because it happened right when I arrived in Israel and not a few days earlier, I believe I picked up the virus in Kenya. There's no way to reverse engineer what happened in my system, so that explanation will have to do. More importantly, I really don't care what happened in the past since it won't change the present. I have diabetes, and I'd better start getting used to it.

Even if we don't know what gave me diabetes, we do know what didn't give me diabetes, and this is perhaps far more impressive based on my penchant to seek out and consume all manners of sugar. The two glasses of chocolate milk I would drink every morning; the boxes of Count Chocula I ate growing up; the orange-mango coolattas from Dunkin' Donuts; the Nesquik powder I would eat with a spoon; the confectioner's sugar I ate from the box; the Lucky Charms marshmallows that I would separate from the flavorless bits and devour by the bowlful; the chocolate bars I destroyed; the pint of Ben & Jerry's ice cream I went through almost every night my first year of college; the chocolate donuts that got me through multiple exam weeks; the sugar-filled carbonated beverages I polished off; the chocolate chip cookies I craved—none of these had anything to do with diabetes. (But they may have had something to do with my root canal.)

Dr. Carracino talks to me about the risks of diabetes—eyesight, nerve damage in the feet, kidney failure, etc.—and then reassures me that, with some discipline, the disease is perfectly manageable.

"My brother has had type 1 diabetes since he was a little kid," he tells me, "and he's doing great. No problems, no complications."

Carracino looks over my blood sugar numbers and my notes. I have a copy of the insulin regimen from Dr. Bhattarai, and he scans that while flipping through the paperwork from the hospitals.

"There's not much I can add to this. You're doing fine. Try to keep your numbers a little more under control, and you'll be fine."

We ask a few questions—my dad, who insisted on being here, chimes in with his own questions—before the appointment is over. As we prepare to leave, Cassie picks up the conversation we started at the hospital in Nepal.

"Once Oren gets better, we were thinking of finishing our trip. How long do you think we should wait before we start traveling again?"

"You can start right now if you want to. You know what you have to do. If your blood sugar is high, take some insulin. If it's low, eat some sugar. There's not much to it. But I think if you wait two months, you'll be ready to go."

"We were thinking four to six weeks?"

"That shouldn't be a problem. Come see me one more time before you leave." With that, we shake hands, and I collect a bewildering array of prescriptions for all sorts of medical paraphernalia that I never needed before. My dad is not happy that we're already talking about getting back on the road.

My prescription list includes the following: Lantus, which is a slow-acting insulin that I take once a day; Humalog, which is a fast-acting insulin that I take before each meal; a blood-sugar monitor; blood test strips to use with the blood-sugar monitor; extra needle tips for the insulin; extra needles to poke my finger and test my blood sugar; and glucagon, an emergency shot in case my blood sugar drops dangerously low. The Lantus and Humalog come in what look like large, disposable pens with replaceable tips. When the insulin runs out, I throw out the pen and use another. (Generally, when I am referring to how much insulin I take with food, it is always the fast-acting insulin. I take sixteen units a day of the slow-acting insulin unless noted otherwise.)

In the US, blood sugar is measured in milligrams/deciliter, or mg/dl. The healthy range is between 80 to 120 mg/dl. Anything below that is hypoglycemia, or low blood sugar. Anything above that is hyperglycemia, or high blood sugar.

It's amazing how quickly I become accustomed to piercing my fragile epidermis with injections at least four times a day and my finger with a sharp, spring-loaded needle before and after every meal to monitor my blood sugar. It takes a week or so, but I soon find it to be routine. As my blood sugar falls back into the healthy range, my eyesight normalizes, and I start injecting myself up with insulin instead of relying on Cassie's help.

One night, Cassie and I go out to a Mexican restaurant with my dad. I order chicken fajitas and try to size up how many tortillas and how much rice I'm going to eat. Generally, I try to take about one unit of insulin for every fifteen grams of carbohydrates in my food. For example, a bagel with sixty grams of carbs would require four units of insulin.

"How much insulin are you taking?" my dad asks.

"Three units," I answer, eyeballing the rice. My dad has to look away as I jab the needle into my stomach.

"Why so much?"

"Each tortilla is one unit, and I think the rice is about one unit."

"Hm."

This becomes a cycle. Every time my dad sees me taking insulin, he has to know how much I am taking. Never once does he say, "I think you should take one or two more units." He always feels I am taking too much. And he is never bashful about offering his advice, even though he doesn't have diabetes and has had no reason to study it until now. He always ends the conversation with a terse "Hm," as if never quite happy with the final result.

A bit of history about the Big D.

Diabetes mellitus was first identified in 1500 BCE by the Egyptians. An Egyptian manuscript described it as a "too great emptying of the urine." Around the same time, Indian physicians noticed the same disease and called it "honey urine" because it attracted ants and flies. This became the first test for identifying diabetes. In 230 BC, Apollonius of Memphis became the first person to use the term *diabetes*. Diabetes is a Greek word, meaning "to pass through." Apollonius thought it was a disease of the kidneys, and his treatments including bloodletting and dehydration, two completely ineffective treatments that did nothing to treat the disease.

Artificial insulin, which is the medicine I inject into the fat around my stomach so frequently, was first invented in the early 1920s. Frederick Grant Banting was a young war veteran and orthopedic surgeon when something about diabetes caught his interest. He worked with his partner, Charles Best, experimenting on pancreatectomized dogs, that is, dogs who have had their pancreas removed, forcing them to instantly develop diabetes. After a number of experiments—and even more diabetic dogs—the two learned that pancreatic extracts injected into the veins of a diabetic dog caused an immediate and dramatic improvement in symptoms. They repeated the experiment on other pancreatectomized dogs with similar results.

On January 11, 1922, Banting and Best injected a fourteen-year-old boy named Leonard Thompson in the buttocks with fifteen cubic centimeters of their extract. Thompson was a patient at Toronto General Hospital who had diabetes. He was down to sixty-four pounds, and his blood sugar was 520 mg/dl. Upon receiving the injection, Thompson became incredibly sick, and abscesses developed on his buttocks. Undeterred, Banting and Best prepared a second, improved injection of their new extract. Thompson's blood glucose dropped to 120 mg/dl, and the ketones disappeared from his urine.

Banting and Best must have been relieved, but not nearly as relieved as the dogs. Their new extract was called insulin.

What is insulin?

Insulin is part of the mechanism that allows the body to absorb fluids and nutrients. Without insulin, my body cannot do anything with the water I drink or the food I eat. Instead, it would all pass through my system instantly, which explains the constant thirst and need to pee. That's why I had to run out into the middle of the freezing Wadi Rum desert to relieve myself. This thirst was the first symptom of my disease. Bereft of calories and nutrition, my body consumed the only protein it could access—my muscles, which explains why I lost an outrageous amount of weight so quickly. I pissed away thirty pounds of muscle. That's what Cassie saw in Israel when she first noticed my weight loss. On the Himalayas hike, the difficult final stretch before Annapurna Base Camp wasn't hard because of my physical condition. It was nearly impossible because I had incredibly low blood sugar, having delayed breakfast until we reached our destination. The second I sat down and had a Coke at the top, I spiked my blood sugar and felt great again. The cramps I experienced on the first day of hiking were the result of dehydration.

The first doctor's instructions to eat more fruit and drink more fruit juice were, in hindsight, both a blessing and a curse. The curse part is obvious. That doctor sent my blood sugar into the stratosphere, accelerating my downward spiral into diabetic ketoacidosis, a very dangerous condition where the body poisons itself. But I see it as a blessing for the exact same reason.

Without his terrible medical advice, I probably would've kept going for a few more weeks without visiting another doctor or hospital. I would've been in bad shape, but not horrible shape, hovering somewhere above the danger zone without plunging straight into it. Because of his general lack of sound medical knowledge, my condition deteriorated so rapidly that I had no choice but to go to the hospital, and that's where I finally got the help I needed (even if it took me two tries to find the right hospital). Once the doctors gave me insulin, I immediately put on weight, through both fluids and solids.

Since then, pharmaceutical companies have cranked out insulin pumps and continuous glucose monitors and insulin pens and inhalable insulin—and the list goes on. Frankly, I don't know whether to be thrilled about all of the medical advancements in the last fifty years or pissed off that no one has cured this disease in 3,500 years, so I politically plant myself somewhere in the middle. I will be content with my disease, thankful that, if treated well, it is a nuisance and nothing more.

What will my life be like from here? It will be just as fun and ridiculous as it always was. To me, there is no old life and new life. There is life. There is no before and after. There is now. Life wasn't ever really normal before, so why should I expect it to become normal?

Let's review: A suburban Jewish kid from New Jersey falls into a career in television news while simultaneously learning to fly a plane his father built in the basement before quitting his job to travel the world with his interfaith wife. Does that storyline change all that dramatically if we add the modifier "diabetic" into there? Don't think so.

I won't ask the question, "Why did this happen to me?" Very simply, it happened. Not everything has to happen for a reason, even though I feel that most things do. It won't help me to sit there and pointlessly ponder if diabetes was part of some bigger plan.

More importantly, it's not fair to others to ask that question. Why did one of my best friends have a stroke at the same age at which I developed diabetes? Why did an acquaintance of mine die in a car crash in our fourth year of college? Why did a friend develop a malignant tumor in her early twenties, forcing her to go through multiple rounds of chemotherapy? These people and their families may ask, "Why did this happen to us?" I have no such right. Not with something as simple and treatable as diabetes.

I know I am not alone.

The World Health Organization estimates that nearly 450 million people around the world have diabetes. In the United States, approximately twenty-nine million people have diabetes. Only about 5 to 10 percent have type 1 diabetes, in which the pancreas simply quits producing insulin. (The vast majority have type 2 diabetes, where the pancreas works, but fat cells get in the way of the insulin doing its job.)

Type 1 diabetes is almost always diagnosed before or right after puberty. It is incredibly rare for type 1 diabetes to happen after age thirty. I guess that makes me lucky.

For those keeping score, that's now two straight misdiagnoses from medical types. After I blew out my knee the previous June, the resident at UPenn hospital said I had probably just strained something. It took my insurance two weeks to approve an MRI because she didn't order one at the hospital that night. And then Dr. Diabetes couldn't figure out that I have the same disease he does. Seriously?! You guys spend eighty-seven years in medical school. Let's make sure your diagnostic accuracy rate is a bit higher than the MLB batting average. Derek Jeter is allowed to bat .310. You are not.

And now, a few quick personal notes.

To the medical staff at CIWEC in Kathmandu: Thank you for getting me home so quickly once my care was in your hands. I think my parents appreciate this even more than I do.

To my pancreas: I'll see you in hell. Quitter.

To Nesquik chocolate milk: I will do everything in my power to work you back into my life in a way that's good for both of us. Right now, we need some time apart. It's not you. It's me. You haven't changed. I have. Our relationship lasted thirty-one amazing years. You'll always be in my heart until you're again in my stomach.

Back at home, I assemble a diabetes travel kit with all my prescriptions and a few other items to help me along the way. I buy a diabetes food guide to gauge how many carbohydrates and sugars are in the food I'm eating, a small digital food scale in case I need to weigh food, measuring cups, and glucose tablets to keep my blood sugar up in case it drops too low.

Although the future suddenly seems very uncertain in ways it didn't just a few weeks ago, Cassie and I are sure of one thing: we want to finish our trip. That may seem crazy. In fact, it may *be* crazy. But for us, and more importantly for me, it's a very simple decision. If I decide to call off the rest of the trip now, then I have already given in. I have accepted restrictions on my life, and that sets a dangerous precedent so soon after my diagnosis. If I limit myself now, I will limit myself forever.

Naturally, my parents completely disagree. My dad wants me home for at least two months ("until Passover"), and my mom wants me to cancel the rest of the trip. We have a very different goal. We want to be on the road again by Cassie's birthday, which is the fifth of April, only a few weeks away. Anything worth saying in an Israeli family (or any other Mediterranean family, from what I understand) is worth saying at 160 decibels, and so we discuss the acceptable date of departure in ways that sound and feel very much like shouting matches.

"You can't leave yet. You're not ready! Traveling with diabetes is different, and you don't know how to do it!"

"Of course it's different! It will always be different! I will never learn how to travel with diabetes while staying at home not traveling with diabetes."

"I want you to stay at home a few more weeks."

"Why?"

"So you can learn more about diabetes."

"What more is there to learn? The doctor said I would be ready to travel."

"The doctor doesn't know you."

"Yes, but you don't actually know anything about diabetes."

And so on and so forth. These arguments continue ad nauseam with no one conceding defeat. We are determined to travel, and my family is determined to convince us otherwise. Finally, Cassie and I decide to buy our tickets without parental approval. We book our tickets—a flight on March 25 to Bangkok via Hong Kong.

When my family sits down to our final dinner together before the flight, I have to count my carbs, shoot up with insulin, then wait five minutes for the medicine to kick in as my family begins eating. It doesn't feel strange around friends or strangers. It does around family for some reason. I suppose it's something I now have a lifetime to get used to.

I eat two bagels, slathered with cream cheese and covered in lox, with a healthy dollop of whitefish salad on the side.

"How much insulin are you taking?" asks my dad.

"Eight units."

"Why so much?"

"Each bagel is four units."

"Hm."

We are home for thirty-one days and a couple of hours. Our flight leaves at two in the morning from Newark airport. This time it's my parents who drop us off at the airport for our flight to Bangkok with a layover in Hong Kong. My dad gives me a bear hug that is just as tight and strong and worried and loving as the one he gave me the moment we landed back in the United States after my diagnosis. He gives me one last piece of advice before we head for the check-in counter.

"At your age, everything should be working. If something isn't working or you don't feel good, come home." It is good advice. I had to come home once; I don't plan on doing it again. All I need is for my body to cooperate, which it hasn't had a great track record of doing lately.

While checking in for our flight to Hong Kong, I see the ticket stub from my last flight—Etihad Airways 101 from Abu Dhabi to JFK on February 21. I am reminded of everywhere I have been—physically and emotionally—over the last five weeks. It makes me hesitate for a long moment. Cassie is making a bit of idle chitchat with the airline employee, so I have time to stare at the small piece of paper tucked into my passport. So much has changed. So much seems fundamentally different than it had when I was on that flight.

Once again, only one thing is certain.

We are on the move again.

Chapter 14

April 6, 2014
20°21'07.0"N 100°04'57.5"E
Chiang Rai, Thailand

I can't quite tell if our tour guide is a guy or a girl. Or maybe a guy who used to be a girl or a girl who wants to be a guy. Such distinctions are often blurred in Thailand for reasons I can't quite pinpoint, and the line between men and women is murky in ways that can be very confusing, as evidenced by Bangkok's lady-boys, a thriving industry of beautiful women who just happen to be men. I have no idea what it is about this country—maybe the food, maybe the heat, maybe fresh fruit shakes that cost two dollars apiece—but changing from a woman to a man (and presumably back again) seems to be no big deal. They have a refreshingly liberal view about sexual identity, even if it makes it somewhat difficult to identify which particular gender you find yourself talking to at any particular moment. Theoretically, the odds of guessing must be fifty-fifty, but I somehow feel far less confident than I statistically should be.

"Our first stop today will be the White Temple," says our guide, whose Adam's apple I didn't notice for the first few hours of our tour. This turns out to be only partially accurate. Our first stop is, in fact, the tourist shops on the way to the White Temple near something advertised as a thermal geyser.

The thermal part is true. There is a thermal spring roughly halfway between Chiang Mai, the largest city in northern Thailand, and Chiang Rai, our destination for the day. The geyser part is a mixture of fantasy and nonsense. A pipe clearly shoots out the hot water, creating the "geyser."

After a fifteen-minute stopover, we're back in the minibus on the way to the White Temple.

Ahhh . . . the White Temple. The entire reason I signed us up for a full day of driving to northern Thailand and back in the first place. I had read about the White Temple, officially known as Wat Rong Khun, while trying to figure out where to pick up our trip. It is, by most accounts, the strangest, weirdest, most bizarre temple in Thailand, a not insignificant feat given the other thirty-three thousand temples in this devoutly Buddhist country.

Wat Rong Khun is a Buddhist temple that, much like its nickname suggests, is blindingly, unabashedly white. From across the street, the temple looks fairly normal, minus the hole it immediately begins burning in your retina from its offensive brightness. It is one part temple and nine parts tourist attraction, mixing religion and pop culture in ways I'm pretty sure should never be mixed. How else do you explain the torso, arms, and head of the Predator, from the 1987 eponymous Arnold Schwarzenegger film, sticking out of the ground? The Batman and Hellraiser busts hanging from a tree? The painting of the X-men, Superman, and Batman flying around and kicking and punching stuff in ways that superheroes should, but probably not in Buddhist temples specifically and religious sites generally? Every white thing here is supposed to be deeply symbolic, with white layer upon white layer of hidden meaning buried within each white detail. And yet, instead of feeling symbolic, the numerous movie, music, and comic references make everything feel more than somewhat commercial. The shopping mall across the street doesn't help.

We have seen hundreds of Buddhist temples since getting back on the road, and they all feel distinctly more—how shall I say?—Buddhist than this one. If there is a deeper meaning here, I haven't quite figured out what it is.

A few months after our visit, an earthquake hits the area and damages the temple, which seems to answer the question "What does Buddha think of this temple?" with little room left for doubt.

For a long time, we debated where we should get back on the road. According to our original plan, we were supposed to splurge on scuba diving lessons in southern Thailand before heading north to explore the more historic part of Thailand. In the end, we decided to cut out the scuba lessons. Something about the possibility of having low blood sugar while sucking compressed air underwater didn't appeal to me.

I blamed myself for the lost time because of diabetes and our time at home, and I promised Cassie we would not cut our trip short again.

We booked a flight to Bangkok via Hong Kong. The airline served a couple of meals, all of which turned out to be breakfast. The twelve-hour time change meant we essentially had an incredibly long day, so we ate breakfast about four times in a row and consumed a commensurate amount of coffee to go with it.

We landed in Bangkok before noon, and it was scorchingly hot. We went from below freezing in New Jersey to a hundred degrees in Thailand. Anyone who says they are a fan of hot weather needs to experience the combination of soaring temperatures and drenching humidity that are a staple of Southeast Asia. You don't so much breathe the air around you as drink it.

It feels good to be back on the road—strange at first, but good. Being back in Bangkok, back at what was supposed to be the next destination of our trip, makes everything seem very surreal. My parents, my family, and my friends are once again thousands of miles away. I rely on Cassie the same way I relied on her throughout my hospital ordeal. She is my sounding board and my emergency plan.

Together we figure out how much insulin to take for meals, what to eat, when to snack, and all of the necessary processes that are now a part of my life. If something goes wrong and I pass out from hypoglycemia, she has a glucagon shot that she'll stick into my leg. It's a huge needle—big enough to throw as a javelin—encased in a bright red box that practically screams "Only for use when the shit hits the fan."

One of my friends asks how it works. I open up the case and show her the needle, filled with a transparent liquid. She half turns away, afraid to even look at something that might draw blood. I remove the three plastic safety caps, two from the needle and one from the vial of powdered medicine I need to mix it with to activate the glucagon.

"Where do you inject it?" she asks, peering cautiously at the syringe.

"Straight into my iris." I jab the needle toward my eye as she defensively posts her outstretched hand between herself and the needle, using the other hand to cover her mouth.

"No, no, it goes into my thigh," I say, trying to reassure her before she gags.

It doesn't take us long to realize that managing blood sugar on the road is a whole new ordeal we have to figure out. We are constantly active, walking all over whatever city we happen to find ourselves in, and we have to deal with the relentless heat on top of that. Over and over again in those first few days, my blood sugar comes in low when I measure it. My plan was to keep my blood sugar higher than normal—somewhere between 120 and 150 instead of between 80 and 120. Not dangerously low, but low enough that it's alarming. My blood sugar is regularly in the mid-80s, which is only about ten points away from where it starts affecting me.

Different people suffer different symptoms from hypoglycemia. If my blood sugar drops too low, my hands start shaking. Gently at first, but if it continues dropping, the shaking is noticeable. As a makeshift way of checking blood sugar, I hold my hand out in front of me to see if it shakes. However, it's not the best way to judge, since low blood sugar can make me a little dizzy, and it becomes hard to focus.

If my blood sugar drops into the danger zone, I start sweating profusely. Not just a few drops of sweat on my brow—every part of me begins to sweat. Sweat stains spread across my shirt; beads of sweat drip off my forehead. Once or twice, it became difficult to talk. I managed to formulate words in my head, but when I tried to vocalize them, the syllables came out all jumbled up.

There have only been a handful of times when I've ever gotten this low, and my immediate reaction is to consume anything around me that contains sugar—cookies, orange juice, Skittles; anything. It's a race between me and my plummeting blood sugar, and to win, I have to eat as much sugar as is humanly possible in about five minutes.

We adjust my insulin levels as often as we have to, but I'm still powering through the Gummy Lifesavers I have as my emergency source of sugar. I buy whatever the local candy is so I always have some form of sugar with me.

At the end of each day, Cassie and I look over my blood sugar numbers. If they all fall in the healthy range, somewhere between 80 and 150, I draw a smiley face in my notebook. In the first few weeks are we back on the road, I stockpile very few smiley faces. But gradually my numbers improve, and my smiley face collection grows.

Bangkok is as exciting and alive as I remember it. The city is a boiling hot cauldron of sights and smells, only some of which I can identify. Street vendors are cooking up all sorts of completely unidentifiable meats, cars are stuck in traffic jams that stretch for miles (or rather, kilometers, now that we're once again somewhere other than America), and the city is bubbling with an urban grit that is awesome to experience, even if it is the second time.

And so I dive into a bowl of spicy seafood soup as our first official lunch on the road. I am punished for my bravery. The food unleashes an inferno of pain on my taste buds, and I expect a similar magmatic sensation after my digestive system does its thing. I take big gulps of water to cool my mouth, which only spreads the spiciness out so it's all over my mouth and lips. Everything hurts. The world hurts. And yet it's so damn tasty. So I keep eating.

I exhaust my table's supply of delicate white napkins that I was using to dry the tears from my eyes and blow my nose. When the napkins run out, I run to the bathroom to use paper towels . . . three separate times. I splash water on my face and eyes, blowing my nose repeatedly to try to expel the conflagration in whatever form possible. The Thai people at the tables surrounding us stare at me. I have reinforced all of their stereotypes about Americans trying to eat Thai food. Without a doubt, I am embarrassing Cassie. Yet, deep down, even with hellfire unleashing the fury of its anger inside my mouth, we are both sublimely happy to be back on the road.

We spend less time outside than we did before. The heat forces my body to burn blood sugar at a stunning rate, so we eat longer meals in air-conditioned restaurants. It costs us a bit more but allows me to learn about my disease before it knocks me out.

We make our way north through Thailand, relying on buses and trains to hopscotch across the country. Our only goal is to reach Chiang Mai, where we spend a week exploring the city and its surroundings, and that includes our day trip to the Chiang Rai region.

From the White Temple, we head to the Golden Triangle, the intersection of the Ruak and Mekong Rivers at the meeting point of northern Thailand, northwestern Laos, and an eastern land peninsula jutting out of Myanmar. The surrounding air bears a cumbersome mixture of searing heat and oppressive humidity. You don't so much feel the weather here as bathe in it. The fervent efforts of our mini tour bus's air conditioner offer only the slightest bit of relief, but under the weight of this weather, any break from the heat is a welcome respite as we shuttle from one tour stop to the next.

At one point, this was one of the largest opium-producing regions in the world, and I'm not sure if that point was five years ago or five minutes ago. Apparently, it wasn't surpassed until the early twenty-first century, when Afghanistan claimed the title. But it feels a bit like this entire area could, in a pinch, once again output fairly impressive quantities of any number of drugs, opium among them, if it isn't doing so already. Historically, they know what products have done well for them, and I'm sure they could produce those products again if they felt any pressing economic need.

Although the opportunities present themselves at multiple points throughout central and northern Thailand, we don't do drugs here. We don't do drugs anywhere for that matter, but there are few places in the world where they are easier to obtain or cheaper to buy than the backpacker-friendly streets of Thai cities and towns.

Travel itself becomes our drug. It is highly addictive and very expensive. It's also stimulating in much the same way I expect cocaine would be, except cocaine wears off while travel does not.

Cassie and I are addicted to traveling.

The effects of travel are also quite the opposite of other drugs. Instead of losing ourselves, we find meaning. Instead of forgetting memories, we remember moments. I can recall almost every day of traveling. Not specific dates or anything like that, but if you ask me about my third day in Dublin, I can tell you about three friends meeting us at our hostel, about the walking tour we gave them, about our first stouts together, and much more. Our second day in Budapest? The Parliament. Our fourth day in Paris? A day trip to Versailles.

It's not that I have some exceptional memory. Quite the opposite, in fact. It's that travel makes the world—your world—exceptional and worth remembering. At my reporting job in Philly, I had trouble remembering the stories I had done the week before. Sometimes even the day before.

On the road, it's absolutely different. Everything is worth remembering. Every sight, taste, and smell is worth hanging on to and cherishing. I remember every day simply because I want to remember every day. Everything is new and exciting and worth permanently etching into my memory.

Once you become accustomed to something, you begin to close yourself off to it. You catalog a set of assumptions and biases about the way
one particular thing works, and you use that information to create what
will eventually become habit. Armed with this routine, you are free to dull
your senses. What you have been through countless times before becomes
uninteresting because of repetition.

Now, our infant eyes are opened wide once again as we take in the
world around us. We open ourselves to places we've never seen and foods
we've never tasted and spices we've never smelled. Our five senses are on
fire, our brain in overdrive trying to store every bit of information for future
recollection. We have not been this accepting of the world around us—this
innocent and naive—since we were children.

It is this incredibly optimistic view of the world that I use to justify trying my first shot of cobra whiskey.

There is nothing subtle or mysterious about the contents of cobra whiskey. Take some awful whiskey, put in a perfectly good poisonous snake,
and drink after it's all commingled nicely together for a few months. The
alcohol is supposed to neutralize the poison while the snake adds a bit of
flavor to the whole affair. That makes it safe to drink, but that doesn't make
it a good idea.

I couldn't resist.

We encounter cobra whiskey in a free trade zone in a section of the
Golden Triangle in Laos. A boat takes us from Thailand, across the river, to
a sprawling gift shop complex in Laos. The free trade zone is the gift shop.
We are not allowed to step one foot out of the gift shop area without the
proper visa, which was not included in our tour package.

Our guide marches us right over to the nearest gift shop and plants
herself (or himself) behind the cobra whiskey.

"Free!" she proclaims with a sense of excitement that is supposed to
entice us to try some, as if anything that doesn't come with a price tag is
automatically worth doing. Perhaps she even wants us to buy a bottle as
a keepsake. I'm pretty sure US Customs would not take kindly to a dead
reptile inside a bottle of alcohol.

She points out the other whiskeys near the cobra whiskey: gecko whiskey, scorpion whiskey, and tiger penis whiskey. The last of these is supposed to be a potent aphrodisiac.

I convince myself that cobra whiskey seems the least harmful. Cassie convinces herself that there is no compelling reason on earth to try cobra whiskey. All evidence to the contrary, I did score higher on my SATs than she did.

I happen to be standing right next to a Canadian guy who seems to share both my age and my reluctance.

"I'll do it if you do it." Of course, that means we're both going to do it.

Our guide pours us a shot of cobra whiskey, and we stare at it for a second, wondering if we're really about to try this.

Of course we are! We have accepted our fate. A final moment of thoughtfulness is all we need.

"Cheers!" We clink glasses and drink.

It tastes . . . not nearly as awful as you would expect it to taste. It certainly doesn't taste good. But it's not horrific, which I consider a win.

Added bonus: I'm still alive.

Chapter 15

April 14, 2014
19°52'44.9"N 102°08'00.9"E
Luang Prabang, Laos

In most countries, it would be considered wildly inappropriate to splash random people with buckets of water as they walk down the street. At best, this would qualify as exceptionally rude. At worst, it is probably punishable by caning in nations with a more conservative ethos. Even in Laos, the transfer of water from a plastic receptacle to someone's clothing is probably not a commonly acceptable thing to do to complete strangers on any given weekday. But our timing in Luang Prabang, the cultural heart of Laos and the country's former capital, is fortuitous. It is Songkan, the Lao New Year, and it is a weeklong party in an otherwise very reserved and quiet city.

Every April, during the hottest time of the year in Southeast Asia, the Lao people come together to celebrate and welcome the upcoming monsoon season and, presumably, break from the ridiculous heat that forces all of us to sweat profusely. As if this isn't enough, we also have to take malaria medication.

The owner of our hostel welcomes us with a big smile and a quiet "Sabadee!" in his delicate, airy voice. He shows us to our room and politely warns us that this is the hottest time of the year.

"For me, is a little hot," he says, fanning his shirt in case we don't intuitively understand the concept of warm weather.

"For you, is very hot." Given the level of heat, this may still qualify as an understatement.

Apparently, the best way to show the monsoons where to unleash their seasonal downpours is to get everyone and everything as wet as possible. Hence the water buckets. Never mind the fact that we are already abundantly moist from sweating through our clothing and that, in having water thrown at us, we were simply replacing our own biological drenching with a more artificial one.

During Songkan, the entire city becomes a free-for-all water fight (as does most of Southeast Asia). Children armed with three-dollar water guns line up along the streets and spray every pedestrian and motorist. Adults use hoses or buckets, but the effect is inevitably the same. One pass through central Luang Prabang and you are soaking wet, regardless of what defense mechanisms you have prepared. After weighing our options, we conclude the best defense is a good offense, so we purchase our own water gun and fire back at anyone who fires at us.

At some point in the last few hundred years, someone must have realized that adding alcohol to a city-wide water fight would neatly complement the festivities and perhaps entice the monsoon season to come just a little sooner to share in the merry-making. Adults, tourists, teenagers, and nearly everyone old enough to hold a bottle is sipping, drinking, chugging, shotgunning, pounding, imbibing, quaffing, or otherwise consuming beer. A sizable majority of the population brave enough to venture outdoors is, without question, happily drunk, and most of those who aren't drunk are well on their way.

Age seems to have little to do with who's drinking and not drinking. Truckloads of barely post-pubescent teens drive around the streets, showing off the beer bottles they have just emptied, inevitably only a moment before they spray you with water. On just about every level, I suspect there is something wrong with the scene around me, yet I have no intention of alerting the authorities, since most of the authorities are part of the scene around me. That . . . and the fact that it's a hell of a party.

Alcohol wasn't the last major addition to change the face of smashing Songkan. With the advent of portable stereo equipment, loud music became an integral element of the already boozy hydro-brawl. Most of the tunes are techno, or at least they sound like techno, though it is admittedly difficult to tell since every volume knob is cranked well past the point of discernible audio. The music pours forth in one mucilaginous mess of noise, which fits in rather well with the prevailing vibe.

There are weird sexual undertones to the entire celebration. Young girls drink bottle after bottle of beer and grind their asses onto young boys' crotches. There is erotic dancing and suggestive singing on every street corner. I suspect a large portion of the young Lao population loses their virginity during these festivals.

What's stunning is how much this differs from their normal demeanor. The people of Laos are humble and gentle and kind in every way. Anger is not something we see a lot of, if at all, and it feels like everyone we see, from waiters to cab drivers, tries to accommodate us in any way possible. Nothing exemplifies this spirit better than the morning procession of monks through the center of Luang Prabang. Every morning, as the sun rises, and the temperature along with it, a long line of Buddhist monks marches silently down the main street, carrying a small cauldron. As they walk, hundreds of people on the sidewalk give them rice or fruits or sweets, placing it right into the cauldron. It will be the monks' only meal of the day.

And yet the monks do not hesitate to give back. Parents or children in need bring their own bowls as they wait along the sidewalk, and the monks dutifully fill the bowls of the needy from what they have just been given.

During this entire process, which can last more than half an hour, no one says a word. The ceremony feels as delicate and fragile and generous as the whole country. In this one morning ritual, you get a sense of the Lao people.

Then Songkan comes and turns everything upside down. This normally quiet society abandons all its norms and goes absolutely hog wild. It is a stunning juxtaposition, as if the Lao population stores its entire reservoir of energy, saving it for one week in April, before letting everything out.

The party settles down at dusk, quelled by a combination of excessive heat and alcohol. The city becomes normal once again, and a sprawling night market opens up where only hours ago a massive water fight raged.

Cassie and I wander around the market for a bit, not particularly interested in buying anything, but always happy to look around and experience the street life. The number of stands selling keychains and home decorations fashioned from unexploded American bombs dating back to the

Vietnam War is more than somewhat disturbing and attests to the distinction Laos holds of being the most bombed country per capita on earth.

It is here that we stumble upon our luckiest find of Southeast Asia, not including mangosteen, two-dollar pad thai, and tiny fish that eat the dead skin off your feet while you sip a cocktail. This year, Songkan coincides with the Jewish holiday of Passover. (That's not the luckiest find. We're getting to that.)

While the Israelites were busy wandering around the desert for forty years (Moses: "Of course we're not lost!"), the Laotians were throwing wild parties and waiting for rain. We would celebrate the Lao New Year during the day and the Jewish holiday at night.

When we landed in Luang Prabang a few days ago, I had plans to celebrate Passover at the local Chabad house. Chabad is a religious Jewish organization with houses all over the world that welcome Jewish travelers, giving them a kosher meal, a bed, and a place to feel comfortable. You can find Chabads almost anywhere, especially across Southeast Asia, where Israelis love to travel.

The only problem with my plan is that Luang Prabang is one of the few major cities in this region that does not have a Chabad house, which is to say, it does not presently have a Chabad house. It did, not all that long ago, and the Web still turns up plenty of sites directing you to 46 Soulignavongsa Road.

But the people who ran the house apparently didn't understand the basic rules of not preaching to visitors and not being too loud about your religion. This is a Communist country, after all. These infractions got the Chabad house kicked out of town some years ago. As someone who hadn't visited a single Chabad location in the eighteen countries we'd already visited, this news shouldn't have been all that disturbing.

Except it was my primary plan for how to celebrate Passover, and I had no backup plan.

It wouldn't be the end of the world if I didn't mark the holiday somehow, but Passover has always been a special holiday to me, and my father's seders—the festive meal at the beginning of the holiday—are not to be missed . . . unless you happen to be traveling halfway around the world. These meals and the ceremony that surrounds them are painfully long. If you do it right, it takes four hours, easy. But if it's done well—and my dad does it very well—they're a hell of a good time.

The longest portion of the meal is reading the story of the Exodus, which takes more than an hour and involves its own unique set of rituals. Much of the story is read out loud, but many parts are sung in their own tune. The problem is that no one agrees on the parts to be sung or the melodies with which to sing them. Half of the meal is spent arguing about what's a song and what's not a song, shouting about the tune of the song, realizing nobody knows the melody and it may not be a song anyway, then trying a number of generic Jewish holiday melodies to see if they fit the words. Inevitably, all of these melodies sound like a depressed alphabet song, and when the vocalist realizes the mistake, the most frequent strategy is to gradually fade out and wrap it all up with a bit of humming.

I knew I wouldn't be able to engage in such lively and spirited arguments with a completely new group of people, but I still wanted to celebrate the holiday. I had pretty much given up on my chances of finding a random group of Israelis wandering around northern Laos—when I suddenly found a random group of Israelis wandering around northern Laos.

When I heard a guy and a girl speaking Hebrew in the aisle next to us in the night market, I charged through the divider of the night market and ran right up to the couple.

"Do you have a place for Passover?" I spewed in Hebrew. Mind you, this is not a standard greeting in Hebrew, or in any other language or culture on earth for that matter.

They were surprisingly calm given my random outburst.

"Yes, we're doing a seder at Spicy Laos," they answered, only mildly alarmed.

"Can I join? I mean, my wife and I."

"Of course!" I can't tell if they agreed because they were legitimately excited to meet new people or if they unwillingly acquiesced for fear of what a raging, Hebrew-speaking lunatic charging through a quiet market was capable of doing should they dare say no.

Regardless, they had new Facebook friends, and we had a place to celebrate my favorite holiday.

We make our way to our festive meal after cleaning up from the day's water fight. We find our new friends on the second-floor balcony of Spicy Laos, one of the cheapest backpacker hostels in the city. A private bunk in a dorm room costs six dollars and comes complete with all of the following amenities: a kitchen, searing heat, drunken screaming from the courtyard, a completely ineffective fan, and a mosquito net. All of our new friends have the slightly sunken eyes of otherwise energetic people who have been forced to endure a few too many nights of inadequate sleep. Most of the dozen or so people are Israeli, but a few are Dutch.

Our extended table is covered in a carefully placed patchwork of banana leaves, providing a sort of placemat for the people seated around us. One of the girls in our group has spread out bananas, rice crackers, a few eggs, and a bit of lettuce on the knee-high table in front of us. A Passover seder has a required list of foods that are supposed to sit in the center of the table. None of what's in front of us comes even close—only the eggs—but finding unleavened bread in Laos was not a task anyone wanted to attempt.

With the exception of the two people we met in the night market two nights ago, we know absolutely no one here, and yet we have committed to spending the entire evening with them, given the importance of the occasion.

We go around the table, introducing ourselves in English so that every-one can understand, before we immediately abandon niceties and conduct the rest of the night entirely in Hebrew.

One of the most important items in the course of a Passover seder is the Haggadah, which is the book that contains the order of the meal and the story of the Exodus. Naturally, no one brought one. Everyone has been backpacking as long as us, and a weighty book that only serves a purpose on one night of the year did not make anyone's packing list.

Someone manages to load the Haggadah on an iPhone—a not insignif-icant feat given the lack of reliable Wi-Fi—and we pass the phone among the Hebrew speakers who each read parts of the story.

Halfway through the meal, a German backpacker sits in the corner next to us, watching our meal while liberally taking hits from his bong.

"Now it's like home," shouts the guy we met in the market. "Except it's this guy smoking instead of Grandpa!"

Since nobody at the hostel is about to whip up a meal for fifteen people, we figure it would be easier to grab street food. After we make it through the story of Passover, we all go out to eat together. I know I will probably never see these people again, but for one night we are our own bizarre little family.

The Passover seder is a perfect way to end our time in Laos, especially since the beginning of our time here almost made me call off the rest of the trip.

When we first arrived in Laos, our hostel owner gave us a city map and showed us where to find food in a small alley right off the night market that he cleverly labeled "Food" on the map.

We found the food alley and ducked inside. Overflowing bowls of seasoned vegetables and rice, flavored with different spices, filled long picnic tables on one side of the tent-covered street. Chairs crammed together around small tables filled the other side, allowing us about eighteen inches of space to make our way down the alley. Most vendors served only vegetarian meals. The ordering process was simple. You paid for a plate, then filled that plate with as much food as you could for a flat fee. The plate cost ten thousand Lao kip, which worked out to $1.25. A few stands had skewered fish or chicken for a few extra dollars. Nothing there appeared to have been prepared within the last twenty-four hours, but we didn't complain, since we were eating only vegetarian, and it was quite delicious. I had broccoli with red seasoning and some broccoli with green seasoning, along with a side of broccoli with yellow seasoning.

My stomach held together for all of about twelve hours.

At breakfast the next morning, I picked at the oranges and eggs.

"Are you okay? You don't look great," Cassie said.

"Yeah, I'm fine," I said, before bolting upstairs and throwing up in the bathroom. I didn't know if it was the food or the malaria medication that we had just started taking, but I was out. Down for the count. I tried to eat a banana and drink some water. That came up too.

Normally, it wouldn't have been that big of a deal that I wasn't able to hold down food for a day or two. But it's a big problem for people with diabetes. A very big problem. If I can't eat, I can't keep my blood sugar up, which puts me in danger of passing out in a country whose medical facilities are probably far closer to Nepal's than I'd like to imagine.

I spent two days in bed while Cassie looked up medical advice and emailed doctors back home.

For the first time since we started traveling again a few weeks ago, I seriously questioned my decision to get back on the road. I didn't have a particularly good handle on my disease yet, and reliable medical help was very,

very far away. Once again, I felt stranded. I couldn't hold back the tears of self-doubt. I cried for a few minutes, collected myself, then cried again. As I lay in bed, trying to feel better—or at the very least, less worse—I kept hearing my dad's words.

"At your age, everything should be working. If something isn't working or you don't feel good, come home."

He was right before, and he was probably right again. Everything should be working. Except something wasn't working, and I wasn't sure what it was.

For two months, I had refused to acknowledge the obvious signs that something was wrong with my system. Now I knew exactly what was wrong, and yet I found myself again trying to convince myself that I was okay. It was déjà vu at its absolute worst.

I tested my blood sugar over and over again, worried that it would drop into the 50s and below. It came back in the 70s. It was a far cry from keeping my blood sugars in the 120 to 150 range. We had the Glucagon shot if my blood sugar dropped dangerously low, but to use it that early in the trip would have been to admit defeat. It would have meant packing our bags and going home. I could already hear my mom and dad lecturing me. This time, there would be no arguing, because they would have been 100 percent right. Maybe I should've stayed home. Maybe I should've called off the rest of the trip. Maybe I should've found a job and returned to a normal routine. Maybe I was wrong . . . again.

I nibbled on granola bars, afraid of taking more than only the smallest bits to avoid upsetting my stomach. Cassie gave me probiotics to see if they would help.

Gradually, I stopped feeling like shit. I could hold down a bit of food, then a few bites, then a full meal. It took nearly three days to recover, and I still felt a bit weak from not eating, but at least I was back where I needed to be. I promised myself this would be the last time I ever shed a tear over diabetes.

My blood sugars were where they needed to be, my stomach wasn't stamping every bit of food with the words "RETURN TO SENDER," and we were on the move once again.

And it felt awesome.

Chapter 16

April 22, 2014
11°34'14.4"N 104°55'47.5"E
Phnom Penh, Cambodia

I never see the bastards coming. There are two—one driving the motorbike and the other sitting behind him. The second guy is the thief. The first is the getaway driver. Their target is a small pouch sticking about two inches out of my left cargo pocket. I'm sure they think it has money since, somehow, I doubt they realize that no tourist would have his billfold hanging out of his pocket. Inside the pouch that I got from Etihad Airways on my way home after my diagnosis are my diabetic supplies: my blood sugar monitor, test strips, and about a third of an insulin pen. The red plaid pouch scores far more points for functionality than style.

They yank the pouch from my pocket as Cassie and I are walking to dinner along the river in Phnom Penh, Cambodia. They make a left and speed off. I immediately start sprinting after them, running full speed for about fifty meters, adrenaline pumping through my veins. Without my diabetes supplies, I am left guessing at my blood sugar. My glucose monitor is the single most important piece of equipment for me to control my diabetes. I cannot imagine a life without it because there is no life without it.

I keep them in sight, but I'm not exactly closing the gap. It's not that I'm slow. Quite the contrary. I was the fastest Jew in my high school, which almost means something since my high school was 40 percent Jewish. I even earned the nickname Jewish Lightning back then. But Usain Boltstein I am not.

I flag down a car and yell at the driver, "Follow that bike!" When the driver speeds off without me, the fruitlessness of the situation dawns on me pretty quickly. Cassie has the presence of mind to flag down a passing motorbike right after I get pickpocketed, and she hops on and puts up chase. As she passes me, she gleans as much information as she can from me.

"What was their license plate number?"

"I don't know!"

"What were they wearing?"

"I don't know!"

"What did they look like?"

"I don't know!"

I always thought I would be so astute if someone succeeded in pickpocketing me. I would know within seconds that something was missing, and I would immediately create a list of suspects from all of the people I had seen within the last few minutes. I would recognize their faces, their clothes, and any distinguishing features. I would pick up on the curly dark hair, the small tattoo of a coiled snake on the back of the neck, the white unlaced shoes, the stained jeans. The suspect would be caught within hours, facing justice and the prosecution I would press to the fullest extent.

None of that happened. I couldn't remember even a single detail. There were two young men on a bike. They looked Asian. And I can't even be sure about that. That's all I've got, and that's probably not enough to launch a police investigation. I had made it through all of Europe's pickpocket danger zones: Paris, Rome, etc. And I get tagged in Phnom Penh, Cambodia.

Phnom freakin' Penh.

I look up and down the street, struggling to catch my breath after my impromptu sprint. To go up the street is to pursue the captors of my supplies, and even I realize how pointless that is; to go down the street is to admit defeat. I was enjoying the relatively cool night air, but now I am sweating again, and not just from exertion. I had never planned for this contingency, never thought there was any way I would let anyone or anything separate me from my monitor. Without my supplies, my heart beats a little faster and my breaths become a little shorter. I was hoping the punks would open the pouch, realize there was no money inside, and throw it to the street, but they aren't kind enough to do that. Instead, Cassie and I shift quickly from the burning desire for vengeance to the pressing need to find a way to keep track of my blood sugar.

We grab a tuk-tuk and go to a couple of pharmacies before we find one that has a blood sugar monitor and test strips. Not the OneTouch device that I had, but a cheap generic brand that seems to work well enough. It costs us forty-two dollars. We spend another twelve dollars on fifty test strips.

Cassie and I come up with a simple plan. Get enough test strips for my replacement device to get me to Hong Kong (about two weeks away), and there I can buy a new OneTouch blood sugar monitor since I'm carrying hundreds of OneTouch test strips. Watson's Pharmacy, one of the biggest chains in Hong Kong, responds very quickly to my customer service email and includes a list of all the OneTouch supplies they carry, which is fantastic. That will be our first stop when we get to Hong Kong.

When we arrive back to our guest house, Cassie explains to the receptionist what happened, while I figure out how to use my new blood sugar monitor, which happens to be quite a bit bigger and bulkier than my old one. The receptionist is so upset she almost starts crying. I find that odd, since I'm the one with the chronic disease, but I will not be the one to ruin this emotional moment.

We try to comfort her, reassuring her that we don't hold it against her or Cambodia. Quite the contrary. We've had an incredible time in her country, and this little incident won't change our opinion.

We spend a day exploring the Killing Fields near Phnom Penh and the Tuol Sleng Genocide Museum in the center of the city. In a very real and heartbreaking way, the Killing Fields represent the Cambodian Holocaust, except the mass slaughter didn't target outsiders, though anyone with a connection to a foreign government or ethnicity was also killed. The slaughter targeted Cambodians. Khmer Rouge leader Pol Pot massacred somewhere between one and four million of his own people in the Cold War era. Walking around the Killing Fields is hauntingly similar to walking around Auschwitz. The voices of the dead cry out to you. Here, there are fewer pictures than at Auschwitz, and all of the torture buildings and prisons that once stood here have been demolished. Instead, fragments of bone jut out of the ground, reminding you of the crimes that took place in these fields. We were warned to look out for bones, especially after a storm, since rain can wash away the top layer of soil and reveal another layer of human remains.

Very often, when Jews speak of the Holocaust, they say "Never Again." Yet it did happen again—maybe not to the Jews, but the systematic slaughter of an entire population took place less than forty years later. The world had not learned its lesson. Pol Pot's Khmer Rouge government held on to the Cambodian seat at the United Nations until 1993, long after the world knew what happened at the Killing Fields.

To summarize my feelings while learning about this part of history, allow me to quote my favorite author, Douglas Adams, from *Last Chance to See*: "Human beings, who are almost unique in having the ability to learn from the experience of others, are also remarkable for their apparent disinclination to do so."

Before coming to the Cambodian capital, Cassie and I spent most of a week in Angkor, visiting the country's most popular tourist sites and marveling at massive stone temples that date back some 1,200 years. The centerpiece of Angkor is Angkor Wat, meaning "Temple City" in Khmer, the native Cambodian language. Angkor Wat is the largest religious monument in the world, covering 1.6 million square meters. Originally built as a Hindu temple in the early twelfth century, it eventually became a Buddhist temple. Today, Angkor Wat draws in more than two million visitors a year, and I think most of them were there on the day we went.

We wake up early to watch the sun rise over Angkor Wat, meeting our tuk-tuk driver at 4:15 in the morning outside our hostel. Tuk-tuks are motorbikes connected to a few seats on wheels, and they serve as cabs in most of Southeast Asia. We are among the first at the temple, and we plant ourselves right next to a small, mosquito-infested pond so that only someone willing to risk malaria will stand in front of us. Then we wait.

Within thirty minutes of our arrival, thousands of tourists are standing around us, filling in every available space with tripods and cameras. Moving is not an option. To give up a spot here is to never return.

The first hints of sunrise come as the sky lightens from black to dark gray to deep blue. Faint oranges seep in at the edges, gradually painting the sky in bright pastels. When the sun creeps above the temple, rays of light burst forward, and the entire sky ignites into a fiery, bright orange. It is absolutely spectacular, and worth every moment of waiting.

From there, we spend the day exploring Angkor's other temples. What's amazing about many of the temples is that you can climb all over them. Very few have any restrictions, and there are no guards or warning signs telling you what to do or where to go. (Angkor Wat has quite a few restrictions, but it's also the most visited, largest, and most famous temple.) The jungle has consumed many of the temples, adding a dark, haunting beauty to the atmosphere. Massive trees grow out of stone towers, the roots snaking their way through cracks and crevasses in stones. One tree has even grown around a stone doorway, giving the distinct impression that centuries passed here without any form of human intervention. If New York City were left alone for enough generations, it would look like a modern version of Angkor, consumed by the wilderness into which it was carved.

One of the most famous temples we visit is called Ta Prohm, better known as the scene of one of the *Tomb Raider* movies, and it is here that we interrupt our story for a moment. Aside from being an incredible temple set deep inside the jungle, Ta Prohm has what creationists claim is undeniable and incontrovertible evidence that evolution is an outright lie and the earth is only a few thousand years old, not the silly 4.5 billion years that every respectable scientist on earth believes. This proof comes in the form of a three-inch carving that looks quite a bit like a stegosaurus.

I have to admit, I didn't see the stegosaurus when we visited the temple because I didn't know it existed until later. But this seems like the kind of off-kilter story that fits right into this book. Had I known about it, I probably would've swapped out the entire diabetes section of this book with a few chapters on this mythical, history-changing, science-crushing, fact-obliterating dinosaur engraving. Why anyone would offer such proof at a Cambodian temple deep within the woods, as opposed to, say, a populated area that can be easily spotted from any direction, has never been made clear.

For those who don't know or have briefly forgotten, stegosaurus was the dinosaur that no one really liked. It was an herbivorous dinosaur that walked on all fours, had protective plates sticking straight up out of its back and running along its spine, and had sharp spikes protruding from its tail. This last bit is about the only cool thing about it. It wasn't as ferocious as a tyrannosaurus rex or as big as a brachiosaurus. Stegosaurus ate low-lying shrubs and bushes, had a very small brain, and lived in what is now the

United States and Portugal, when the two were smashed together on earth's one mega-continent a few million years ago.

The stegosaurus carving is near one of the many doorways at Ta Prohm, about five feet off the ground, surrounded by intricate portrayals of other animals, decorations, and vegetation. By general consensus, it is not a fake. Back when Ta Prohm was being built sometime in the late twelfth century, its builders carved a stegosaurus into its facade.

"Aha!" says the skeptical sleuth. He mulls his evidence over once again before proclaiming it to the world, making sure it all checks out.

"Aha!" he repeats. "If people who built this a few hundred years ago knew what a stegosaurus looked like and how to carve one, then dinosaurs must have been around a few hundred years ago. The artist must have seen a stegosaurus in person!"

He pauses a moment, collecting his thoughts and making sure they are in all order before proceeding to the grand crescendo.

"And if dinosaurs were around a few hundred years ago, then clearly evolution is a lie, fossils are fake, and creationism is the only plausible explanation." He concludes his argument, cooing loudly to show his self-satisfaction to the world, clearly unable to detect his own putrid nonsense. There are a number of websites that support this exact argument, though I will not, for your sake, point you to any of them. Suffice it to say that the Internet isn't always right.

Fundamentalists of all shapes and sizes seize on this hapless stegosaurus. "God created all the land animals and man on the same day! So says the Bible! Therefore, dinosaurs and man must have lived together in perfect peace and harmony."

The argument is bulletproof, and any rebuttals that the carving also resembles a rhino in front of some vegetation, or that there are plenty of mythical carvings around Ta Prohm, or that stegosaurus remains haven't been found anywhere even remotely close to Cambodia are misguided falsehoods that merely bounce off the ironclad logic of the faithful. Apparently, the stegosaurus is carved out of solid bullshit, completely impervious to the weathering of storms, time, and common sense.

No, clearly, whatever determined artist carved this here illustration decided that this would be the one spot where he would leave absolute proof that he once caught sight of a stegosaurus while going for his daily stroll. Science and fossils be damned. And just to make his point, the artist carved an animal that looks an awful lot like the Cheshire cat a few inches below the stegosaurus. Clearly, that must have existed too, and presumably this is the spot where Lewis Carroll found his inspiration.

This bit of nonsensical trivia makes me enjoy the Angkor temples in general and Ta Prohm specifically even more. I prefer my wondrous archaeological sites mixed in with a healthy dollop of wild conspiracy theories, and the fact that there are few other such sites connected to said theories is something I'm sure the new-earth creationists will soon rectify, hopefully in time for my next round-the-world adventure.

As we leave Ta Prohm, sans pictures of our ancient reptilian quadruped but with about a hundred other pictures of us climbing all over the temple, we stop for a fresh coconut. Every temple has its own well-armed militia of coconut salesmen. They wield sharpened machetes, ready to violently and efficiently thwack the top off a coconut for one dollar. (The official Cambodian currency is the riel. Since roughly 4,000 riel equals one US dollar, Cambodians prefer dollars. They will occasionally give you change in riel, so that if you buy something for $1.75, they will give you the equivalent of 1,000 riel instead of 25 cents, instantly making your change worthless. Although they're happy to get rid of riel, they're loath to accept them back.)

The coconuts, of which we purchase quite a few in our attempts to quell the palm fruit warriors, offer a quick and healthy boost of sugar in the blazing heat of Cambodia. Temperatures rarely drop below ninety degrees, so I'm always sweating and always burning through blood sugar. The coconuts are a quick fix.

At one point toward the end of a day at Angkor, we can't find a coconut vendor, so we buy a Coke. I have a few sips to keep my blood sugar up. As of this writing, this is the last sip of Coke I have had. It's strange the things you take note of after a diabetes diagnosis.

And while we're on the subject of blood sugar, one last thought on the jerks who stole my blood sugar monitor.

Over the last few months, I've had to look at a lot of different things in a positive light, and this is no exception. I consider it a win-win situation that they got away. Those two punks didn't have their arms broken, and I didn't have to go to a Cambodian jail. Given the generally fervent belief in karma in this part of the world, I fully expect they will develop type 1 diabetes.

In that case, I hope they held on to the monitor, since it's a damn good one.

Chapter 17

April 24, 2014
10°46′34.2″N 106°41′40.1″E
Saigon, Vietnam

Ho Chi Minh City, or Saigon as most people here still call it, is exactly as crazy and hectic as we've been told. Motorbikes seem to spawn and multiply in real time, so that if you see one down the street headed your way, it becomes 12 by the time it reaches you, then 50, then 137, each blasting its horn in a chaotic symphony of noise that might as well be the Vietnamese Philharmonic Orchestra, because the musicians on their two-wheel hell-riders play it all the time.

The high-pitched whine of the 125cc bikes are the sopranos, the six-cylinder Toyotas and Hondas are the altos, and the trucks with their clank-clanking rumble fill in the bass and percussion. Saigon has life, all right, unless that life inadvertently steps in front of a bus. By the looks of the streets, the unfortunate meeting of flesh and fender should be happening all the time, but there is the slightest hint of coordination on the roads, and our friends explain the simple rules of surviving as a pedestrian.

"Just start walking across the road. The motorbikes will miss you. Don't cross in front of a car or bus. They won't stop."

From what I can tell, the best preparation for crossing the street in Saigon is to play Frogger on an old Atari until your eyes bleed. No amount of planning or strategizing better simulates the streets of the city than the 1981 console game, in which you must guide a frog across five lanes of alternating traffic and a river, which somehow also has five lanes. The cars come at you from all different directions at all different speeds, and to survive you must choose when to move with traffic, against traffic, and when to stay put. The game might as well have been called "Frogger: Streets of Saigon."

As in most of Southeast Asia, lane markings, traffic lights, and anything that might imbue a sense of order are mere suggestions to be promptly ignored if inconvenient. I never see anything that might be a speed limit. Cars and motorbikes and buses pick their own speed in a way that appears quite random. What amazes me is the only rule that everyone seems to follow. If you break one traffic law, you have to break them all. No one *only* speeds. You speed, weave, fail to use turn signals, drive the wrong way down one-way streets, park illegally, and have a broken headlight all at the same time.

Even on the five-hour bus ride here from Phnom Penh, sometimes we would go fast, sometimes slow, without any discernible relation to the condition of the road, the velocity of other traffic, or our surroundings. Why does the left lane go fast, the right lane slow, the right-middle lane somewhere between moderately fast and decently slow, and the left-middle lane at a ludicrous speed? Maybe Saigon's Director of Public Development had an Atari 2600. It would explain a lot. Saigon makes Bangkok look like a quiet city.

Our guest house is a ten-minute walk from the bus stop, during which at least fifty cab drivers, motorbikes, and bicycles with attached chairs ask us if we need a ride. Apparently, there is a law covering all of Asia that requires everyone to bombard you with questions and requests as soon as you step off your bus or plane. Maybe it's some sort of ingratiation ceremony, in which case I'm not showing nearly enough deference and respect for the local custom. Or maybe it's a sort of hazing to prepare us for what's ahead. If so, I dread what's ahead.

Our street is twenty feet wide with thirty feet worth of stuff packed into it—street vendors and people and bars and cars and, of course, motorbikes. Our room on the fourth floor keeps most of the noise out, but there is a constant drone of activity that is perpetually audible. It is the white noise of Saigon. Having worked our way through three countries in Southeast Asia already, we are mentally and emotionally prepared for the cacophony.

It is insane in a way cities that grew up too fast always are. Too many people, not enough development. Still, it is fun to walk around.

The soaring temperature hasn't even considered abating yet, so a five-minute walk at night leaves us drenched in sweat as if we had just completed back-to-back marathons. We expect cooler temperatures in North Vietnam. We just don't know how far north we have to go to notice any real difference.

We visit the Vietnam War museum in Saigon, known as the War Remnants Museum, which gives us a very different perspective on a war we didn't learn enough about in high school. Though any museum with a wing called "Historic Truths" must be approached with a bit of skepticism, we enjoy our visit, and learn just how terrible Agent Orange was, which was noticeably lacking from our grade-school education.

After two nights in Saigon, we fly to the center of the country, visiting Hoi An and Hue. Our final stop before Hanoi in northern Vietnam is Phong Nha, home to what was the largest cave in the world before they discovered an even larger cave nearby. We rent motorbikes and explore the area with some Dutch friends we meet at our farmstay. Without knowing it, our stay here coincides with one of the biggest holidays of the year in Vietnam—Reunification Day, also known as Victory Day or Liberation Day. On April 30, 1975, North and South Vietnam were united and the Vietnam War officially ended. To celebrate, many Vietnamese visit the exact cave system we're visiting, which means the lines are long and the waits even longer, but with nowhere to be and nothing else on our agenda for Phong Nha, we enjoy ourselves and our new friends.

The owner of our farmstay, an Australian guy who left all of his worries Down Under, books us an overnight sleeper to Hanoi for the last leg of our Vietnam wanderings, and after one night in Phong Nha, we bid adieu to the farmstay and the neighbor's cow, who walked over to say goodbye. A transfer bus takes us to the café that serves as the bus station for the sleeper bus.

The sum total of all the white people on our sleeper bus is four: the two of us and the Dutch couple.

We have heard horror stories about the sleeper bus from pretty much everyone who has ever taken it, known someone who has taken it, has thought about taking it, known someone who has thought about taking it, or has ever been on a bus before. It isn't a sleeper bus at all. A sleeper bus implies that you can actually get some sleep, which numerous online reviews and travelers claim is absolutely impossible due in no small part to the ongoing disco music played at unreasonably high levels and the abundance of fluorescent lights that are never turned off, no matter the time or how many hours remain until sunrise and our arrival at our stated destination.

EdwardRY from Beaumont kindly informs TripAdvisor that the sleeper bus is not the most pleasant experience. "It's nothing short of hell. Should have taken the train, or did we actually drive on the RR tracks all the way? . . . The driver hammers on the horn continually. Music on the speakers until 1 a.m. No shocks on the Huong Long red bus—or maybe even tires. Driver thinks he's on a moto, swerving and braking and stopping for a whiz every 20 miles like my kids! And you sleep on dirty sheets that are still warm from the last body—ugh!"

YorkFoodie: "As has been pointed out, you are more likely to arrive in one piece if you take the train: besides the insane traffic and poor roads, some buses are driven by absolute cowboys who may even be . . . er . . . chemically enhanced, which does not improve their driving skills."

The last review is much shorter and to the point, though somewhat less colorful. "Sleeper buses are an unforgettable experience, and one never to be repeated."

So it is with a healthy amount of trepidation that we four foreigners step onto the bus. If I am going to die, this is as good a time as any. The young Vietnamese usher immediately herds us to the back of the bus. He speaks not a word of English, but strangely enough is fluent in German, which does me no good since that's not a country we visited on our trip. Even if we had, I'm pretty sure my German vocabulary would have been limited to *yes, no, cheers,* and *weinerschnitzel,* so I'm not sure how much progress we would have made.

Every Vietnamese person gets their own reclining seat on the bus, but only one of our small team of foreigners gets an individual bed—the Dutch girl. The rest of us have to share the only communal bed on the bus, way at the back, as far away from as many people on the bus as possible. I get the sneaking suspicion this is more for their convenience than for ours. And so it is that I end up in the middle, Cassie on my left and our Dutch friend, Marc, on my right—a *ménage à trois* of travelers on an overnight bus to Hanoi. We play involuntary footsie for most of the ten-hour bus ride, gently intertwining big toes and caressing feet because our sleeping arrangement leaves us no choice.

I don't understand any of the words uttered by the Vietnamese people looking back at us, but I can imagine their phrases roughly translate to "Suckers!" or "Stupid white people!" or "This is what they get for bombing the shit out of this country."

Conveniently, we are next to the toilet, which inconveniently means that whenever someone goes to relieve himself or herself, our auditory and olfactory senses are promptly and duly notified.

Our bus sets off at about 8 p.m. and makes its first stop at about 8:05 p.m. I'm not quite sure what's happening since the only thing I can see from my elevated perch at the back of the bus is three square meters of the ceiling. All I know is that we're stopped for a long time, at least twenty minutes. At this rate—20 percent driving and 80 percent stopping—we are not going to get to Hanoi before our flight to Hong Kong in six days.

Cassie, who has a window seat offering her a slightly better view, says they are packing the storage compartment of the bus with cargo. I wonder whether it's of the rice variety or the opium variety. Neither would particularly surprise me, but at least I now understand why they threw our backpacks on the beds below us instead of the luggage hold.

The bus sets off again and maintains what feels like a pretty good pace judging from the rhythmic rocking of the bus. Left and right. Up and down. The staccato blasts of the horn indicate that we're regularly passing people, so at least we are making something that resembles progress.

And then we stop.

Again, less than an hour into our overnight bus ride, I'm beginning to see the truth in all of the online reviews we have read. This is the bus from hell. I half expect to see our bus driver doing blow any minute. Maybe he'll at least have the common courtesy to pass it around. I've never done cocaine—or any other drug that's not alcohol or the occasional cigar for that matter—but an overnight sleeper bus to North Vietnam sandwiched between my wife and a Dutch tourist who was a complete stranger thirty-six hours ago feels like the right place to try these sorts of things.

Before I get a chance to ask my wife her opinion on my impending drug use, the bus pulls out once again, sans cocaine. This time, we go and keep going. The karst mountains of Vietnam zip by us in the dark. The South China Sea is to our right; the endless rice fields of the countryside to our left.

Much to my surprise, we don't stop again, and remain in a state of fairly perpetual motion until we pull into Hanoi. Contrary to all of the terrifying online reports, the ride was quite pleasant once we got past the first hour or so. We didn't quite make any friends on the bus, but we didn't lose our lives, and that seems like a fair trade.

For the first time in eight weeks, the temperature has finally dropped into the normal range. Days are in the low eighties; nights are in the sixties. No more of the relentless heat of Southeast Asia. I get a better handle on my blood sugar numbers and fall into a rhythm with my insulin. Where previously my blood sugar was dropping below 100 fairly often—a bit too low for comfort when I'm far away from help—now it's coming in around 110 and above. That gives me a bigger margin of error in case something goes wrong or I miscalculate my insulin badly.

We spend five nights in Hanoi, including an overnight trip to Halong Bay—not so much because there are five nights' worth of things to do in Hanoi, but because a four-star hotel costs twenty dollars a night, breakfast included, and we need a break. Hanoi is the polar opposite of Saigon in many ways. It is quiet and ancient and spread out. Nothing seems too urgent, no one moves too fast, and we walk around the beautiful city, drinking *bia hoi*—Vietnamese street beer brewed daily that costs twenty-five cents a glass—while soaking in the culture and the sites.

One night while looking for something new to eat, we settle on a Mexican restaurant, even though we are about as far from Mexico as you can get in Hanoi and we should've learned our lesson the last time we ate Mexican food in Poland. At least the weather is nicer this time, the mood is brighter, and the margaritas are made with tequila. We sit on the second floor balcony, enjoying some generically Tex-Mex staples like burritos and sipping our sweet and tangy drinks. The only thing better than one margarita is two margaritas.

Big mistake.

Two hours later I check my blood sugar. 271. Officially my highest blood sugar since I began taking insulin. My second favorite mixed drink—

dirty martini is my favorite—is off-limits from now on. Lesson learned. Two units of insulin and my blood sugar comes down into the normal range. There will be no smiley face in my notebook today.

Cassie and I retreat to our hotel room, where we while away the evening hours sending emails, sorting through pictures, and relaxing. I realize Cassie has something she wants to say, and yet she is hesitant to say it. Having now traveled halfway around the world and been through a life-changing diagnosis together, this immediately strikes me as odd.

She opens her mouth, then closes it. A moment's pause.

"Do you regret traveling?" she asks.

Cassie doesn't mean getting back on the road. She means getting on the road in the first place. If I had somehow known that I would be diagnosed with diabetes on the trip, would I have opted to stay home? Would I have avoided the risks of the road for the comforts and safety of home? Would I trade the life I have now for the life I had before? We have given up our apartment, our jobs, and most of our savings. We are far away from our friends and our family. When we return to the United States, we will have no readily available prospects for employment, no place to live, and no source of income. On top of all that, I have a chronic disease that requires constant monitoring, and we will have to find a way to pay for insurance almost immediately upon our return.

That's what she means when she asks, "Do you regret traveling?" Cassie's question will define how we view this trip.

I have no need to hesitate when I answer. "Absolutely not. I would never trade in this trip for anything, even with diabetes. It may take us a while to find a job and a place to live. I may have to work at a coffee shop to pay the rent. Maybe we'll have to live with our parents for a bit. Doesn't matter. It's totally worth it."

The things that make up a "normal" life—job, home, car, daily routine—will work themselves out. We will find jobs as we once did, and then we'll find a place to live, and we'll go from there. Everything else will work itself out eventually. There is no doubt it will be frustrating, but in no way does that make traveling a bad idea.

And it's certainly not something I will ever regret. I have not yet wrapped my head around diabetes, and I have plenty of highs and lows throughout the course of a week, but I am slowly learning each day. Yet none of that—none of the injections and blood sugar checks—keeps me from enjoying every moment of every day. It will take a bit more time, but I am coming to terms with my disease.

Chapter 18

May 8, 2014
22°20′01.9″N 114°09′47.9″E
Hong Kong

There are few things more enjoyable in a foreign city than finding a local market, purchasing a few morsels of local food, and eating outside on a public bench while absorbing the city's ambience and atmosphere via cultural and culinary osmosis. In Marseille, we bought a baguette, a wedge of cheese, and a few apples for four euros, and enjoyed a perfect meal by the harbor. We attempt the same sort of bare-bones, inexpensive meal on our first full day in Hong Kong, heading to the International Financial Centre mall, which is supposed to have a boutique supermarket and a beautiful rooftop view of Victoria Harbour.

We grab the cheapest bottle of wine we can find—at twenty-two dollars, this is the most expensive cheapest bottle we've come across—and head for the roof garden with a small brick of blue cheese and brie, some French bread, and Italian salami. A meal that cost us seven dollars in France somehow costs us fifty-two dollars in Hong Kong.

We gorge on our "budget" meal. We have no utensils, so in this most cosmopolitan of cities, I tear into the salami with my teeth, biting off hunks and chewing loudly. I imagine the people sitting around us feel like they are the first generation of homo sapiens, curiously looking at the end of homo erectus, hoping that I die off so they can rule the world in relative civility. I suspect they wonder where this savage came from. Philadelphia, bitches! And if you think I'm bad, wait 'til you see what the rest of the city has in store. Everything we lack in major sports trophies we make up for in attitude.

I am afraid to speak, knowing Cassie is angry at me for misfiring so badly on lunch. Much as I hate to admit it, she has every reason to be peeved. I was in charge of procuring a cheap lunch, and the money I spent on one meal could've fed us for two days.

I need to digress for a moment. I wish I remembered the following conversation better, because it has two of the most important quotes from our trip, both from Cassie. When she said these two sentences—and they were not said consecutively—I immediately pulled out my pen and pad and wrote them down. The problem is that I forget what came before or after these sentences, so they only exist in my memory as completely disjointed phrases. Apparently, nothing I said mattered because I didn't write it down, and any and all meaningful thoughts in this conversation—and most others for that matter—came from Cassie.

Here are the two things Cassie said:

"You light a fire and you can't put it out—the idea of traveling."

"It changes who you are. You can try to change that, but you can't."

The people who set out from Philadelphia nearly a year ago were us in name only. We have seen more of the world than we ever thought we would see. We have made friends from countries I barely knew existed. We may not see them again for years—we may not ever see them again—but we have travel in common, which means we will always be able to pick up where we left off. When we go home, we will have changed in ways we never could have predicted, and we will be eternally thankful for that. And for all we have seen, we know there is so much more that we have not seen. Only when you try to explore the world do you begin to understand how truly large it is and how many different stories each little bit of it holds.

As we finish our meal, the first few drops of rain pelt us from above, sending us inside to find cover. It doesn't stop raining for the next four days, gathering in intensity throughout the evening hours until it qualifies as an all-out storm.

We haven't seen rain like this since we started traveling—only the spastic bursts of storms in Kenya and Chiang Mai and the on-again-off-again rain of Ireland that is as much a part of the country as Guinness and whiskey. But, even there, the rain let up eventually.

There are no signs of a respite here from the endless precipitation. The downpour may ease for a few minutes, but it returns with a meteorological vengeance, announcing its newfound energy with staccato explosions of thunder and vicious stilettos of lightning. We knew these days would come eventually; we knew that, statistically, we weren't getting a year of good weather. In all our months of traveling, we had lucked out. Until now.

The rain confines us to our room on the fifth floor of the Mei Ho House Youth Hostel—which, for all intents and purposes, is a hotel, especially in terms of price—and the dining room downstairs. Only a few hours into our climatic prison sentence, we are already going a bit stir-crazy. I can't bear the thought of sitting behind a desk at whatever job I find back home, where we'll be all too soon. That, too, seems like a prison sentence, only it's one imposed by society, not weather.

We venture out only to see the remains of a World War II fort called Stanley Fort on Hong Kong Island. The Japanese attacked Hong Kong the same day they attacked Pearl Harbor. Sort of. The attack happened within hours of the first wave hitting Pearl Harbor, but because of the different time zones and the location of the international date line somewhere in the middle of the Pacific, it was already December 8 when the Japanese attacked Hong Kong. Known as the Battle of Hong Kong, the city held out for more than two weeks before falling to the Japanese army. It would be one of the first battles of the Pacific war. Somehow, my high school textbooks failed to mention any of this.

My Gore-Tex jacket and Adidas shoes, already pushed to the brink months ago in the Himalayas, give out in the ceaseless rain. To be fair, when Adidas and North Face designed our gear, I don't think they intended for it to be dragged around the world, worn every day, and smushed into a backpack for extended periods of time.

Despite the weather, we also venture out to find what I have been missing since Cambodia: a blood sugar monitor that works with all of the diabetes supplies I already have. I know that Watson's, the pharmacy chain here, has exactly what I'm looking for. We find the nearest one on the map and walk in with a premature sense of relief. Watson's has exactly what we need, except it doesn't measure what we need it to measure in the units we want it to measure it in. Since my diagnosis, I have measured my diabetes in milligrams per deciliter, which is supposed to be between 80 and 120. As I find out very quickly, they use a different unit of measurement for blood sugar in this part of the world. Of course, it is one that I have never heard of.

The millimolar.

The millimolar is a measure of molar concentration, and it is generally used to measure the amount of solute in a solution. From high school, I remember that one mole is 6.02×10^{23}, and that's about all I ever intend to remember about moles. Even though the conversion from one unit to the other isn't all that difficult, I make the determined decision to keep using my generic brand blood sugar monitor until I can find one that works exactly like my first monitor did, including the same unit of measurement. Millimolars be damned.

During the brief moments when the rain abates, we can see Victoria Harbour from Mount Davis, a mountain at the western end of Hong Kong Island. We see a traffic jam of ships waiting to enter. And we see storms building all around us. Across the water, Lantau Island is visible, and then it isn't, consumed by the wispy whiteness of a distant storm. From here, it looks peaceful, but in that storm, it's raining like hell.

We take the Star Ferry across the harbor to Kowloon and find a street stall selling curry fish balls, one of Hong Kong's indigenous foods. I order a small bowl using a few frantic pointing and eating gestures I make up on the spot. Cassie refuses to touch the curry fish balls. The balls have the texture of gefilte fish—which is, in some strange Jewish way, oddly comforting— and the seasoning and flavor of Indian curry, making it the strangest commingling of flavor and texture I have ever tried. Some foods are fantastic, others are disgusting, but they are uniformly fantastic or uniformly disgusting. Not Cantonese food. It's great with a slight twist of strange, excellent with a hint of bizarre, or flavorful with a dab of I-can't-believe-anyone-on-this-planet-would-even-consider-eating-this, which is a taste they're quite adept at in Asia, at least to my delicate Western palate.

Hong Kong strikes me as very Dickensian. Not so much in a "best of times, worst of times" way; it is in the extremes here. The city is ultra-modern, yet it hangs on to its roots with its people and its vibrant street culture. A mile away from our hostel, I could find fifty people who spoke perfect English in a heartbeat. Here in Sham Shui Po, I can barely find a menu in English, and Cassie and I resort to pointing at pictures of food to order. That, to me, is the miracle of Hong Kong. It has not lost any of its own culture as it has become an international financial hub. It may have spots that are entirely Westernized, but for each of these spots, there is something that is entirely Cantonese—a place where you would absolutely struggle to understand where you are, why you're there, how you got there, and where you're going next without a firm grip on one of the world's most difficult languages. We know because we found quite a few of these places in our exploration of Hong Kong.

I can't fully explain why I love this city so much. Maybe it's the combination of modernity and tradition. Maybe it's the bizarre street food. Or maybe it's the awesome Bruce Lee statue by the harbor. Either way, I put Hong Kong high on my list of places to visit again. After four days, it is time to make our way north into mainland China.

We had read about the vaunted punctuality of the Chinese train system. Every train leaves on time and arrives on time following its on-time journey that makes all of the intermediate stops on time. After the wild guesswork that goes into the trains in Southeast Asia, we are thrilled to be reading timetables and schedules that are in English and predictable. Cleanliness would be an added bonus.

We arrive an hour early for our train—the T100 express to Shanghai— only to find out that it's delayed. The term *express* is a bit of a misnomer. The train takes twenty-one hours to get from Hong Kong to Shanghai. The only "express" part is that it doesn't make any stops. Twenty-one hours of perpetual motion through the vastness of the Chinese countryside. But here in the waiting area, there is no movement. The train before ours is delayed as well, so a seething mass of passengers destined for two different cities fills a waiting area designed for one train's worth of people.

All the seats in the waiting area are full, so I sit cross-legged on the ground near a pile of our stuff. Cassie stands next to me. There's no point in moving—no point in anything but waiting patiently—but the locals push and jostle their way to the front of the line, itself just a large group with no discernible shape or order huddled near the boarding gate. Their efforts are pointless—both trains have assigned seats. Elevator music plays over the loudspeakers, which seems cruelly ironic because elevators move faster than us at this moment.

The music, which seems like it was carefully picked following multiple focus group sessions, was probably designed to placate the masses. It makes me confident that, somewhere, there is a Chinese ticket agent delivering soma to the unsuspecting. But instead of calming us, the crowd grows restless. All of us are eager to get to our next destination. Every few minutes, the music cuts out and a voice starts speaking in Cantonese. I wait for the English translation, hoping it will carry some news about our train, but the message only repeats the same two warnings: watch out for pickpockets and don't buy counterfeit goods. I find the latter warning to be very odd, since I'm pretty sure 85 percent of Asia's street economy is built on the buying and selling of fake Rolexes and Breitlings. The industry term here is *imitation*. It's not a rip-off Bulova, it's an imitation Bulova. Either way, it looks damn good and will only set you back thirty dollars if you're good at haggling.

The train before ours is cancelled, and the dormant mass of passengers comes to life in a very animated and pissed-off way. The departure board announces the train has been cancelled because of inclement weather. Passengers can get a refund or reschedule at the ticket counter. That doesn't bode at all well for our train, which I'm sure is about to be cancelled. Passengers screaming in both Mandarin and Cantonese rush to the ticket counter. Cassie and I wait for the announcement about our train, but it never comes.

Two hours after our train was supposed to leave, the company hands out free water and crackers in an attempt to assuage our growing annoyance and impatience. After a few more hours of waiting, the train company provides us dinner in another attempt to keep us from storming the ticket counter. Rice and chicken. As simple as it gets. Only, instead of serving us chicken breast or chicken wings or chicken thighs, they serve us cross-sections of chicken. Although this is perfectly normal for the Chinese, it is quite stunning to us, especially in our frazzled, tired state. It is as if someone took a hacksaw across a complete chicken, cutting through skin and meat and bone, and plopped a one-inch section of chicken on a bed of rice. In fact, this is precisely what has happened.

I take a few bites, trying to figure out how the locals around me make it look so easy, but Cassie demurs. This is simply not the dinner we had in mind. Not insignificantly, my diabetes food guide offers little advice on how much insulin to take for one crosswise inch of chicken.

I want to explain to the ticket salesman that I would very much prefer not to be on the first train out of this station, especially given the reports of mudslides and heavy rains across our route. I would much rather be on the second train out, once I know the first train has arrived safely, but I feel like such subtlety would not be fully appreciated. Instead, I get ready to spend the first night of my life in a train station.

It almost comes to that. It is 10:15 p.m. before we finally board, a seven-hour delay for a train system that's supposed to always be on time. More than a few passengers are pissed off when security refuses to let them leave the station. The ticket agents are more determined to get us to Shanghai than we are determined to get to Shanghai. Finally, after forty-five more minutes of waiting on the tracks, the train pulls out.

The train can best be described as completely unremarkable—twenty-one hours from Hong Kong to Shanghai (plus that seven-hour delay, but who's counting?), and there is barely anything worth writing about the journey. We share our six-person compartment with two other people— both Chinese. One speaks no English. The other speaks great English and gives us pointers about what to see in Shanghai and Beijing. As miserable as the wait was, the ride isn't too bad or too good. It just *is*.

The only thing noteworthy about the train—and about the rest of China for that matter—is the prevalence of smoking. No one smokes in our compartment (although I'm pretty sure it's allowed). Everyone smokes at one end of the train car or the other. Whatever end of our speeding locomotive they choose, the stench of smoke fills the cabin. The Chinese have taken to smoking like Michael Phelps took to swimming. They're very good at it, and they do it a lot. I can't imagine what sort of competition they're trying to win with their nonstop inhale-pause-exhale routine, but I conclude there must be one, because only that would reasonably explain how often they smoke and how many cigarettes they avail themselves of. A lot is made about the smog problem in Beijing and some of the other cities in China. I think the reason the Chinese don't care about it is because they've already subjected their lungs to the medical equivalent of drinking tar.

We pull into Shanghai late in the evening, and the first two items on our agenda are finding our hostel and a place to eat. I am glad to be off the train, even if we only have thirty-six hours until we get back on a train for a bullet run to Beijing.

Conveniently, our hostel is on top of a dumpling house, so we order chicken and vegetable dumplings before the restaurant closes. When it becomes obvious they want us to leave, I ask the receptionist at our hostel how to say *to-go box* so we can take the rest to our room.

"*Tow po*," she tells me.

"All I have to do is say *tow po* and they will understand?"

"Yes." Well, this seems simple enough.

I walk the few feet back into the restaurant.

"*Tow po*," I declare confidently in my newly acquired Mandarin.

The hostess shakes her head at me.

"*Tow po*." This time, I try to indicate that all I want is a small box in which to put my food.

Another head shake.

"*Tow po*," I try one more time, with the exact same result.

I conclude there is only one option left. We steal the plate, the dumpling sauce, and the silverware from the restaurant, and head to our room for the evening. The dumplings are quite tasty, with that extra bit of flavor that only petty thievery can impart. We leave the plate in our room for the hostel cleaning staff.

Our explorations begin the next day. We walk along the Riverside Promenade, visit the Old City of Nanshi, and stroll through Fuxing Park. After a few hours of wandering around, I come to one depressing conclusion.

Shanghai is sterile. The Chinese have modernized any semblance of culture out of the city, placing all of the history into one museum, which we don't visit. If they can't be bothered to care about their past, neither can we. Shanghai is one shopping mall after another. There is nothing uniquely "Chinese" to see here. Even the buildings that look historic are only mockups to lure in tourists for another round of kitschy souvenir purchases. The only vaguely traditional thing the city is known for is the food.

Shanghai is famous for dumplings, especially soup dumplings—a delicious little morsel of pork or shrimp inside a steamed dough wrapper that also encapsulates a few flavorful drops of soup. We visit the renowned soup dumpling restaurant, Din Tai Fung, which we fittingly find on the second floor of a shopping mall.

This seems to fit right in with what I know about Shanghai so far.

Oh, and Shanghai's most famous soup dumpling restaurant is a chain from Taiwan. That gives you an idea of the extent to which this city has sacrificed every shred of its five thousand years of culture and history, replacing it instead with glitzy skyscrapers and high-end stores. The city lacks its own character. It is completely devoid of its own feeling. There's even a place here called Shanghai Times Square, which shows you how much this city wants to shed its own identity and subsume the personalities and identities of every other city. As if to exaggerate the point, near Shanghai Times Square is Hong Kong Plaza.

In the evening, we meet friends in Shanghai. Marc and Camille are both teachers at an international school in the city. As with most of the people we meet on the road, our first encounters were through social media. They want to go to Kenya as they embark on their own round-the-world trip, and we had just been there.

"You got lucky," Marc tells us.

"Why is that?"

"The pollution isn't bad today. Normally it's awful. You can't see more than twenty meters. When it's over two hundred, we wear masks."

I'm not quite sure what unit of measurement he's referring to when he says two hundred, but the tone of voice makes it clear that two hundred is such an astronomically high number that we should live in constant fear of it. Terrorist attacks, plane crashes, and the number two hundred. If you have a healthy fear of those three things, you'll lead a safe life.

Marc and Camille take us out to a Sichuan restaurant, and they both impress us with their knowledge of the Chinese language, which clearly exceeds my "tow po."

"Don't be too amazed," Marc tells me. "All I really said was *this* and *that* while pointing at the menu. That's it. It's enough to order food."

We order too many drinks at dinner, then we grab a bottle of wine and head back to our hostel for a few more drinks.

We wake up early the next morning to catch the bullet train to Beijing. Another unremarkable ride, except for the elderly man seven feet to my right who coughs up phlegm every three minutes. I'm no expert, but I would say he probably smokes too much.

Chapter 19

May 15, 2014
40°26′25.7″N 116°31′29.4″E
Great Wall of China

The only problem with the piece of Sichuan rabbit leg I'm eating is that it is not, in fact, a Sichuan rabbit leg. It is indeed Sichuan cuisine, based on the burning sensation in my mouth and the name of the restaurant, cleverly called "Sichuan." And it is rabbit, judging by the consistency of the meat. But it is not the *leg* of the rabbit, per se.

A few days ago, we came to this same restaurant with our friends who speak Mandarin. One of the delicious dishes they ordered on our behalf was Sichuan rabbit leg. It came out on a long, rectangular white plate with five or six rabbit legs lined up in an orderly row, smothered in a spicy brown sauce. The food was so good that we decided to return, and I tried to order the exact same dish because it was so damn tasty.

I get the rabbit part right. But as I flip my piece of rabbit over in my hand, I realize that my rabbit leg has teeth. Either I have been served a mutant rabbit that had teeth on its leg or I have mistakenly ordered rabbit head. That would explain why my dish looks entirely different than the serving of rabbit leg from before. This time, two pieces of rabbit "leg" are served on a circular white dish, and they are symmetrical. My rabbit has had its head cut straight down the middle, with each half of the head facing up, so as to appear more aesthetically pleasing. A closer examination of my rabbit head reveals eye sockets and what I'm pretty sure is the brain. Determined to stick to my rule of eating anything the locals eat, I finish my rabbit head and move on to the dish of spicy cucumbers, which is equally delightful and slightly more palatable.

Sadly (at least if you're picturing Bugs Bunny here, it's probably sad), rabbit head is not the most bizarre food I eat while in China. Take your pick: duck tongue, chicken feet, squid jerky, and a few others I choose not to remember. These foods are as alien to us as General Tso's chicken is to Chinese people. Frankly, I consider this their loss, since General Tso's chicken is delicious. It just has nothing to do with authentic Chinese food.

However, we didn't come to China to eat. We certainly didn't come here *not* to eat, regardless of how many strange and un-Western food–like substances they put in front of us, but food was not our primary goal here. I will shamelessly admit that in China, we came to be tourists. And that means going to the Great Wall.

We wanted to do the Great Wall differently. Most tourists who sign up for a trip to the Great Wall inevitably find their way to one of two different places: Mutianyu or Badaling. These two sections are fully restored, and they are crammed with tourists and vendors selling to those tourists. There is little that is historic or original about what you see. But because these two places are relatively easy to get to from Beijing, they end up being the most common trips to the Wall. We were looking for something a little more authentic. And by "authentic," I mean "illegal." To be fair, I didn't *mean* to mean illegal. It just kinda turned out that way.

We signed up for a three-day, two-night hike along the Great Wall. It promised one night on the Wall and one night in a village near the Wall.

The trip carries added significance for me. There are no hospitals near the Wall, so this hike will be my first chance to push myself since my diagnosis with no nearby options in case of an emergency. This is by no means a strenuous hike—at least it's not supposed to be—but it marks our first bit of serious athletic activity since we started traveling again.

Our tour company tells us to find a guy named Tony at a certain place at a certain time. Just be there; he will find us. Befitting this set of instructions, we meet Tony near the Pearl Market, one of Beijing's biggest counterfeit goods supercenters. He is not a counterfeit goods expert—at least I don't think he is. But he is an experienced tour guide in his early thirties.

Tony is not his real name. Tony is his American name, because my American mouth can't properly pronounce his real name. He has a thick crop of black hair—standard, it seems, for every male in China—and speaks excellent, if slightly accented, English. Tony leads us to a convenience store to grab some snacks, then on to a series of buses and cab rides that take up most of the morning. He keeps pointing at a printed piece of paper he's holding.

"This is what the instructions say to do."

It is comforting that he has instructions; it is equally discomforting that this seems to be the first time he's looking at them.

A few hours later, we pull into a small village that seems a world away from the metropolis of the city, and, after a quick briefing, we head for the Wall.

This is where the "illegal" part of this excursion comes in. It is, without question, against the law to hike on parts of the Wall that are not properly restored, maintained, and sanctioned by the Chinese government. It is also, without question, a very popular undertaking for visitors not content with a simple day trip.

As we approach the spot where Tony intends for us to climb up onto the Wall, a group of locals blocks our path. They demand payment for us to pass. A toll of sorts or, more accurately, a bribe. I have to admire their entrepreneurial spirit and their understanding of the finer points of economics. They have found something in low supply, i.e., entrances to the Great Wall, and decided to charge money for it. Tony is not as amused. He argues with them in Mandarin for a few minutes, but even I realize how fruitless this entire exercise is. We can't report them for illegally charging us for what we illegally want to do. For either one of us to call the police on the other means we will all be thrown out together, and that seems counterproductive for everyone.

We walk for a few more minutes near the Wall before finding a much less hospitable spot to climb up. We're on a part of the Wall known as Jiankou, a secluded, crumbling section that has not been restored, and this becomes apparent as we begin hiking.

There is no smooth, polished walkway down the center of the Wall, and there are certainly no handrails or handicap-accessible ramps. The Wall is falling apart here in very obvious and dangerous ways. This place would've been condemned in the States. Here you just get a warning to be careful. You're on your own. Good luck. Break a leg, but only figuratively.

The disrepair makes the Wall that much more haunting and beautiful. At times, we are not hiking along the Wall—we are climbing. Hand-over-hand scaling. The kind that has very bad results if you fall backwards or misplace a foot, hoping that the next stone is at least as secure as the last one. Cassie, who has some issues with heights, has to pause more than once to collect herself. I see the hiking as a big "fuck you" to diabetes, and I try to move a little faster with a bit more confidence. I will live my life by my own rules and no one else's. I scale back a bit on my long-term insulin to make sure my blood sugar doesn't drop too fast on the hike.

The last time we hiked like this was in the Himalayas, where I probably came closer to dying than ever before. Now I am the master of my disease, not the other way around. It feels good to be healthy, happy, and traveling. I delight in every step and every breath. This is what life is about. Drawing the most out of every moment. Too often, that is an aspiration. Today, it is an accomplishment.

Our host shows up at 6:45 p.m., sweating and exhausted from the hour hike to this point, weighed down by two tents, three sleeping bags, and dinner. Before starting our hike, we had arranged to meet him at an ancient guard tower that predates America by a few centuries. He makes us coffee first—a jolt of warmth as the sun sets and the temperature drops. Then tea. And finally, he puts out a dinner of rice, cabbage, tomato and noodles, beer, and Pringles. The food—quite delicious, especially given how far we are from the nearest kitchen stove—is almost entirely irrelevant. We are eating dinner on top of a tower on the Great Wall of China. He could've served us dog's testicles, and it would've been fantastic.

Our host, whose name we never learn, looks to be in his late fifties, with the same crop of short black hair and the weathered lines of someone who has lived in the country their entire life. And yet his smile comes easily. If he has lived a hard life, he will not let it show. He doesn't speak a word of English, and yet we find ourselves laughing and chatting as we eat. He responds to our "Cheers!" with his "Gan bay!" and we sip our beer as dusk nears. After dinner, he packs up his belongings and heads back down to his village. We will see him again at breakfast.

If the Wall is majestic during the day, it is mysterious at night. We set up camp inside the same guard tower. Small villages surround the base of the mountain we're on. In the distance, the lights of Beijing reflect off of the clouds. The Wall snakes away from us in both directions—we are at the top of a mountain, so either way is down. Only the wind interrupts the complete silence, adding a chill to an otherwise beautiful evening.

On a section of Wall we had hiked hours earlier, we can see the lights from another group bedding down for the night. Out here—out on the Great Wall of China—it's impossible to be anything but happy and at peace. I am in the middle of the world's most populous country, and there isn't a soul around to bother me.

Me, my notebook, and my camera.

In this moment, everything else is superfluous. We travel for moments like this. We *live* for moments like this. Not a care in the world. I shiver against the evening cold, but I don't fret about my lack of a jacket, mostly because I have no choice, having left mine in Beijing. Up here, everything feels like it's far off in the distance. Even Cassie, sleeping a few feet away, feels a world apart. Noises from the villages below are faint echoes, drifting lazily up the mountain to my cozy spot on the Wall. Lights from the towns and cities are nothing more than remote pinpricks of color. I stare into the distance, trying to see as far as I can. Somewhere out there, thousands of miles away, is my home. My family and friends. The life I once knew. We are now just about halfway around the world. Up until this point, to keep going east was to go farther away from where we had come from, and now it is to draw closer. From this point on, every step forward is a step closer to where we started. In a sense, we are at the beginning of our journey home. And yet this feels like where we belong. Maybe not an abandoned guard tower on the Great Wall of China. But this perpetual motion across the earth.

If the night lacks anything, it is a bottle of scotch, and I make a note to include that on my next visit.

It was impossible to think a moment like this was even somewhat plausible when we had started planning our trip. We knew we would see the Great Wall; we just had no idea we would see it like this. Yet here we are, enjoying the quiet solitude of camping, but doing it on one of the Seven Wonders of the World.

No one ever thinks "I'll grab some shut-eye on the Pyramids" or "Let me take a nap in the Colosseum." Those thoughts are absolutely ridiculous and would get you arrested posthaste. But here in China? Totally doable, especially when you have about five thousand miles to pick your spot. I wouldn't say it's exactly encouraged. After all, this is supposed to be a closed part of the Wall, and there are clearly signs prohibiting a camping excursion, but these are at most mere suggestions, which can be liberally ignored, much like traffic laws in Saigon, so long as you respect the Wall and don't break anything that's not your own leg.

This made it absolutely worth everything we went through to get my visa to enter China.

We had been warned that it was not a simple process, so we at least wanted that process to occur in the United States in English so that we might have a fighting chance if we had to enter negotiations. Applying for our Chinese visas in Vietnam seemed rather unwise.

Our first trip to the consulate in New York City lasted all of about three minutes. Cassie had prepared all of our paperwork, checked and double-checked that we had passport photos, itineraries, names and addresses of hotels, and just about every piece of personal info apart from our social security numbers.

The young woman at Window Seven looked at Cassie's application, asked a couple of questions, then accepted the packet with a polite "Thank you."

My turn. Everything was going swimmingly until the woman at Window Seven saw the "J" word on my application. Journalist. That led to an instant rejection and an afternoon of frustration. Cassie's application was retro-rejected.

I had to get a letter from my boss saying the trip was for personal reasons. It was fruitless to explain that I was leaving my job in a couple weeks and would be unemployed, so of course the trip was for personal reasons. I didn't think I'd have any luck pointing out that I cover shootings in North Philly, not international news. I did what in hindsight was the smart thing to do at that point and kept my mouth shut. For this, I applaud myself and my frail sense of patience, for it is at times like this that I tend to become a bit of a misanthrope.

My boss wrote me the letter, confirming that my trip to China was not a professional trip, and I made my second trip to the consulate. This time, they accepted both of our applications and told us to return in a week.

We were optimistic when we went back for our third trip. We had everything lined up and our paperwork was accurately filled out. Turns out only half of us should've been optimistic. Cassie's Chinese visa was approved without a problem. She paid her $140 and got her passport back. I immediately knew something was wrong when I saw my entire application folded not-at-all neatly into my passport. On it, someone had written, "Come back one or two months before entry."

"Why was I rejected?" I asked in a tone of voice meant to hide my growing disdain for the bureaucracy that was driving me nuts.

"Because you are a journalist. Come back a month before your trip to China and apply again," said the supervisor behind Window One, who was quickly becoming the target of all of my negative thoughts.

Before I could fire off a not-so-pleasant response, Cassie chimed in, "We'll be in Cambodia or Laos a month before China, and we want to get our Chinese visa here in the US."

"But you are a journalist. You can't get a visa right now."

I pointed him to the letter from my boss that we had submitted, making it clear that I was leaving my job and that the trip was not professional in any way. Two things became immediately obvious. First, he hadn't read the letter. Nor had anyone else. Second, he realized I was not, in fact, a threat and that I should probably be allowed into China.

He smiled. "Come back after you leave your job and write 'Unemployed.' Then it will be okay."

Nothing about that makes sense. The Chinese would prefer unemployed vagrants to employed journalists? Apparently, yes. And wouldn't the first question from the woman behind Window Seven or her equivalent be, "What was your last job? Oh, journalist? Well, you need a letter that says . . ."

Since I had nothing to lose, we gave it a shot. Four days after I left my job (and two days after we shoved all of our earthly belongings into storage), I went back to New York City alone (trip number four). While I was on my way into the city, Cassie checked online to make sure the Consulate was open. Much to my chagrin, it was open. Much to my horror, they had suddenly redone all of their application forms and stated in no uncertain terms that the old forms would no longer be accepted. Cassie filled out the entire new application for me while I was driving, sent it to me, and I took it in.

Four days later, I went back to the consulate for my fifth trip. Against all odds, they approved my application, and a fairly large, very conspicuous Chinese visa occupied the first page in my passport. As one of my friends put it: Bear Jew: 1, China: 0. I pointed out that it's more accurate to say: Bear Jew: 1 China: 4. It's the 1 that counts.

It took us another nine months, but we finally took full advantage of our visas. And I am absolutely glad that we did.

Long after I should've been asleep in our private little guard tower, I turn in, enjoying the solitude of the evening and the absolute wonder of the experience, knowing I will sleep well tonight after the day's hike. In that regard, I am correct. For all of about two hours.

I suppose it was statistically impossible that our tour guide was the only person in all of China who knew about this guard tower and considered it an excellent place to bed down for the evening. I just hoped whoever knew about the tower wasn't intending to use it on this specific night.

Just before midnight, two people arrive at the guard tower, making the kind of racket fifty campers would make if they banged all their pots and pans together at once. They haven't seen us yet, or at least I'm pretty sure they haven't seen us because I haven't seen the beam of a flashlight, and they certainly assume they're alone based on the cacophony of noise they're creating. It briefly occurs to me that they may be here to rob us, but that notion is quickly dispelled when I poke my head out of the tent and realize they are as surprised to see us as we are to see them.

Attempting to initiate communication at this point would be futile. I don't speak a word of Mandarin (Tony taught me to count to ten earlier in the day, but my accent is horrible and a display of my numerical dexterity would only serve to convince them that I am, in fact, some kind of idiot), and they probably don't speak a word of English. We all arrive at the same conclusion independently. It is best for us to completely ignore each other and for them to find their own spot to sleep somewhere else in the guard tower. In the morning when we go our separate ways, we can all pretend this was a bad dream. I suspect this is much how the first meeting between humans and aliens will go.

I succeed in getting a few more hours of sleep until a heavily equipped group of Chinese cameramen show up at four in the morning to shoot the sunrise. At this point, I concede that the best course of action is to wake up and take more pictures. Sleep will come later.

Our host shows up in the morning and whips up a small but delicious breakfast before we get moving again. He is quickly becoming my hero, with the greatest superpower of all: the ability to make decent food any-where in the world.

After breakfast, we start hiking again. We quickly approach the part of the Wall that is refurbished. After a day of hiking along an original, crum-bling section of the Wall, this seems somehow inauthentic. We divert to Bei Gou, the village where we spend our second night.

Our hostel, a cozy, family-owned set of rooms just off the main road in a town that can best be described as adorable, is empty, save for us. Tony learns from the owners that they have just suffered a loss in the family, and they have been closed for a few days. We offer to find a different place to stay for the evening, but they insist we stay with them.

The owner fires up a small grill and throws all kinds of different skewers on the coals—some of which I can identify, some of which remain a mys-tery to even the most knowledgeable and experienced of culinary minds. They are all absolutely delicious. Lamb, chicken, mystery meat, vegetables, fish, and mystery substance (which may be mystery meat number two, I can't tell)—everything is grilled to juicy, flavorful perfection.

"How is it you speak English so well?" I ask Tony.

"I learn from tourists. Almost all of the tourists speak English."

"Where else do they come from?"

"I have tourists from Israel." He counts to ten in Hebrew, which abso-lutely impresses me. "And Japan. I don't speak Japanese, but we use the same symbols. I could write my messages, and they understand." There is a deep and significant lesson in linguistics here that I'm sure could be used to draw parallels between different people from different countries, if only I knew enough about linguistics to draw it.

"Do you always work for the same company?"

"No. They call me when they need me."

"Why not start your own company? You could advertise on Facebook."

"I have a Facebook account. I checked it once . . . in Abu Dhabi. I was translating for a group of Chinese businessmen. I cannot check Facebook here in China." Tony shrugs.

Up until now, we have only seen China at the inherently shallow level of tourists. This isn't a knock against casual tourism; it is the reality of the experience. You see something, you take pictures, you move on. Now, sitting across from Tony in a village that few Westerners have ever heard of, we *live* China.

We drink round after round of Yanjing beer, having switched away from the horrific 2009 vintage Rove Ruby red wine, which instantly and unequivocally wins the award for worst wine of the trip, usurping the title from the wine we drank in Vietnam and not challenged again until the fermented grape beverage of Peru. Our host keeps churning out grilled mystery skewers, his hospitality unending.

We turn in early. Tomorrow, it's back to Beijing, the big city, but not before a bike tour of our small town. There, we stumble upon perhaps my favorite part of this village. Outside the town's Communist party head-quarters, there is a series of photographs of different villagers who have received various accolades. We spot a picture of our hostel owner's wife on the sign. She has been named "Best Mother-in-Law in Bei Gou."

Chapter 20

May 19, 2014
39°54'46.0"N 116°23'51.2"E
Beijing, China

By my math, I took somewhere north of sixteen thousand pictures during our entire trip. Most of these I promptly deleted, especially since I never take one picture of something—I take four and pick the best one. Yet in all of those pictures I took, I rarely appear. Cassie yelled at me constantly for not taking enough pictures of us, and I have to admit she was absolutely right. But the universe inherently seeks its own balance, and even if I don't have pictures of me, others do.

We arrive in Beijing and navigate the subway to Andingmen, a neighborhood in China's capital that we know nothing about other than that it has a hostel with a private room at a suitable price. Once we leave the subway station, we immediately become completely lost. The hostel is on a street we cannot pronounce, and we are also on a street we cannot pronounce, which makes it virtually impossible to successfully navigate from one street to another, especially since all of the other intervening streets have names we cannot pronounce.

With the conviction of people who passionately believe that everything will find a way to work itself out, we decide to purposefully and determinedly set off in one direction. The specific direction isn't particularly important. What's important is that we have faith in that direction, and a solid belief that it will lead us somewhere and that we will make the best of that somewhere.

We end up on a street corner not unlike the street corner we left. It is the intersection of a major road and an alley. There are a few shops on both sides of the street, and people are generally milling about on what is otherwise a perfectly normal afternoon in Beijing. The only thing that stands out is us. Everyone else clearly knows where they are and what they are doing. We have no such information at the moment.

Having picked up a local SIM card in Shanghai, I dial the number of a friend whom I haven't seen for more than a few seconds at a time since my college years at the University of Virginia. In a city big enough to hold twenty-two million people, Adam is somehow only a few blocks away from us. He instructs us not to move. He will come to us.

As we settle upon a direction in which to stare in anticipation of Adam's arrival, a middle-aged Chinese woman pushing a stroller pauses across the street and looks at us for a moment. I don't know what she's contemplating, but it involves us in ways I cannot quite fathom. She is clearly not going to ask us for directions, since it's obvious we're the ones in need of direction. And she probably doesn't speak English, so it's not worth attempting to initiate conversation.

Instead, she pushes her baby stroller over to us and leaves it there. With the baby inside. She then walks back across the street, pulls out her cell phone, and starts snapping pictures of us. After ripping off a few shots, she runs back over, grabs the stroller (with the baby) and keeps moving. It takes me a second to realize what has just happened.

We had been warned of this. White people aren't all that common in China, not even in Beijing, which has a regular stream of Western tourists. And although I am not exceptionally tall, I am tall enough to stand out in China. Any time we are out in public, people snap photos of us. This happened to us once in Vietnam, but it is a never-ending photo shoot in China. We could choose to resist. We could yell at people for snapping photos of us and angrily shake our fists at them while we scream words they don't understand. Or we could have fun with it. Every time we see someone taking a photo of us, we give them a big smile and a thumbs up. A few times, when the aspiring photographer walks right up to us, we pose for selfies. There's nothing wrong with enjoying our newfound celebrity status, and it balances out the lack of photos of us in our personal camera. At least someone else has them.

A few moments after our first photo experience, I spot Adam. Adam and I worked together at the local AM radio station in college. He took me out on my first story, helped me write it, and taught me how to work the audio board so I could record my voice. I thought he was a few years older than me, until our boss told me he was in his final summer break before college. We worked together for two years at the station, and Adam was always willing to help me out or cover a shift. We got to know each other over long late nights at the radio station while working on different pieces and lamenting about the old dude in the office who never went home and who, rumor had it, had never in his life left his hometown of Charlottes-ville, Virginia. We lost touch after college—I went into news, he managed restaurants—until I heard that he had upped and moved to China.

This did not seem like an Adam thing to do. Adam is a white American Jewish kid from Virginia, with skin so pale it leaves no doubt that he is abso-lutely and completely Caucasian. He doesn't speak another language, he's a bit scrawny, and he never struck me as the truly adventurous type. He was defi-nitely fun, but not crazy. Back in college, he sported a mop of short blond hair to go with a high, nasally voice. If something was funny, he didn't continually laugh. He gave one forceful "HA!" that relied on quality, not quantity.

As Adam approaches, I can see that little has changed. He has the same build, the same hair, and the same smile. Since I haven't seen him in years, I missed the entire age progression from young college grad to working adult. All of the same features, just matured a bit. It is as if police used one of those age progression techniques for finding missing kids.

"It's the smog. When I moved here, I was twenty-five and looked eight-een. Now I'm twenty-seven and look forty." He shrugs.

Above all, Adam looks relaxed. He is wearing a flannel shirt with the top three buttons undone. His hair sticks out from under a woven beanie, and, as it becomes obvious a moment later, he smokes. It is, without ques-tion, awesome to see Adam, and I politely ignore Cassie for a few moments while we bear-hug each other.

He takes us to our hostel to drop off our stuff, and we find our way to a pub where we grab a few beers and sit outside on what is a clear and beau-tiful day in Beijing. We ask about life in China—is it expensive, how's the food, how's the nightlife—and he asks about our trip—where we've been, what we've seen, what was our favorite part.

"We have an obligation to travel," Adam declares with the humorous confidence that feels like it deserves a slap on the back and some spilled beer on our shirts.

"Why is that?"

"Because right now is the greatest time to be alive. In history! Before or after. It's easier to travel now than it's ever been before. And with all the countries opening up, it's all Westernizing so fast. Now—right now!—is the best time to travel."

In my opinion (and if you've gotten this far in the book you must be at least somewhat interested in my opinion), Adam is absolutely right. I can buy a plane ticket from the nearest airport and get virtually anywhere in the world within twenty-four hours or so. If there are layovers involved, forty-eight hours at the most. We have no excuse not to see the world.

We can create excuses if we want. We can meet someone via video chat or see the world through pictures and websites. We can take advantage of the technology at our fingertips to learn so much about so many places. And yet these are half-measures at best. The rest of the world is closer than it's ever been before, and we have a right to see it. It is up to us to exercise that right.

Eventually, our conversation turns to beer, as it often does. I immediately inform Adam that I am a huge fan of India Pale Ales. Adam's eyes light up.

"Follow me."

Adam leads us down a few of Beijing's alleys—called *butongs*—until we walk into a small, dark, dank bar. This is, without question, a dive bar. The beer options are written in chalk on the board, and even though I don't recognize any Chinese symbols, I know enough to know that the owner's handwriting is awful.

"Don't worry about that. I'll order for you."

According to Adam, the owner is one of the best local beermakers, a student of the guru of Chinese microbrewing, an industry I didn't know existed until a few moments ago.

"Two Catbird Asses." I give Adam a look that is meant to say, "What in the name of all that is holy did you just order?" He gets the message and gives me a reassuring "Trust me," which is not at all reassuring. Cassie, wisely, orders soda.

The owner brings us two pints of beer and smiles at me. The beer—a light golden brown—turns out to be an excellent India Pale Ale.

"This guy set out to make an IPA like Dogfish Head 90 Minute IPA," Adam explains, mentioning my favorite IPA on the planet.

"He came damn close!"

"Yes he did. So he figured China is the opposite of America, so the opposite of Dogfish Head is Catbird Ass." Adam clinks my glass and we keep drinking. Sometimes the world makes a tremendous amount of sense, and sometimes it makes no sense at all. This is one of those times where I'm not sure which one it is.

The next day, we explore Beijing, first on a bike tour (our guide asks us if we would like Kentucky Fried Chicken for lunch or a local dumpling house and is clearly surprised when we pick the latter) and then with J. J., Cassie's friend from graduate school at the University of Delaware where the two of them studied English as a Second Language together. J. J. isn't her real name, but it is the closest English approximation to her native Chinese name, so she uses it with Americans.

I can't help but notice that J. J. looks stunningly Western when we meet her in the subway station for Tiananmen Square. She is dressed in a slim black skirt that matches her jet-black hair. Cassie is surprised, and so am I. The last time I saw J. J. a few years ago, she came to our place in Delaware looking like a young student. Now she looks like a confident adult woman.

We aimlessly wander around Tiananmen Square as Cassie and J. J. catch up. I stay a few feet back, taking pictures every few minutes. J. J. is shocked and patently offended when a Chinese family asks to take pictures of us. We tell her it's okay, and then we all smile together, flashing our ubiquitous thumbs up.

As we venture toward the Forbidden City, which is across the street from Tiananmen Square, we see police activity in front us. No surprise here. We are two weeks away from the twenty-fifth anniversary of the Tiananmen Square Massacre. The government has already started blocking websites that make any reference to June 4. A friend tells us that some websites have instead referred to the day as May 35 to avoid censorship. That's a great solution, until the censors get wise to that too.

Most Chinese have only the vaguest notion of what happened on that day. Some people died, they'll tell you. A few criminals. Foreigners, right? No big deal.

There's no point in arguing or trying to explain otherwise, since they've been taught from day one that nothing really happened. Except something did happen. Something really awful that should be mandatory for everyone to learn about, not only here in China, but everywhere else.

During the early months of 1989, student-led popular demonstrations filled Tiananmen Square and the streets around it. This is the cultural and political center of China, akin to the National Mall in Washington, DC, or Parliament in London. Many of the important government buildings are on the street that runs between Tiananmen Square and the Forbidden City, which was China's imperial palace for five hundred years. (Now it is a beautiful tourist attraction in the heart of the city.)

The protesters pushed for liberal reforms in the political and economic systems. In response, the Chinese government instituted military law. On June 4, tanks and troops rolled into the area around Tiananmen Square. The protesters weren't just kicked out. They were destroyed. Hundreds of protesters were killed, perhaps even thousands. The official party line was that nothing major happened back on that day.

But as we get closer to the police officers, we see that something very real has just happened on *this* day. A half-dozen uniformed officers are standing near an ambulance. Another fifteen to twenty men are holding black umbrellas open and pointed sideways, as if it were raining from the left or the right, not from above. Adam had told us the undercover officers would be everywhere in the coming weeks. Now, they're trying to hide something with those umbrellas. Intentionally blocking our view. What is it?

I can't see . . .okay . . . I see a bit . . . it's . . . it's a body.

A middle-aged Chinese man is laid out on the ground. Judging by the blood everywhere and the gauze over his neck, someone cut his throat. There's a 5 percent chance someone had told him not to move so he wouldn't exacerbate the bleeding, which leaves a 95 percent chance that he's already dead. I've seen enough dead bodies as a journalist to know he was killed ten minutes ago at most.

J. J. is shocked. She keeps her cool and knows to keep walking, since everyone else is doing the exact same thing, but a moment later she is visibly shaken. Bodies on streets are not something one comes across very often in China, especially not right in front of the Forbidden City.

The officers—both undercover and uniformed—are moving everyone along. Only one person has a camera out, and he's probably with the police. No one else dares. I have already put my camera away and locked the bag, or else I would try to snap a few quick photos as we walk by. It would be far too conspicuous to undo the lock on my bag, pull out my camera, take off the lens cap, and hit the shutter release button. As I had told the Chinese consulate in New York nearly a year ago, I am not working as a journalist. I am unemployed. Getting thrown in a Chinese prison ranks lower on my list of things to do than spending a week in a Nepali hospital.

But what is plainly visible to me is plainly visible to everyone else, even if they are exercising a certain amount of willful ignorance. A day after seeing the body, I write about it in my little green notepad, and there it stayed until I copied my notes down into this chapter.

The body is gone within two minutes. Police put the guy on a stretcher, get him in the ambulance (or, as we've just learned, the hearse disguised as an ambulance), and remove any evidence that something happened. Anybody who comes thirty seconds after us will have no idea anything was amiss. The general public will never know there was a dead guy near one of their most important national sites—the equivalent of someone getting killed on the steps of the US Capitol. If that happened, it would be texted, Tweeted, Facebooked, Tumblred, Stumbleuponed, Triberred, Reddited, Foursquared, selfied, Pinterested, Google Plussed, and in every other possible way broadcast to everyone in the country. It would make national news. Possibly international news.

Here it has been swept away, and no one will ever know except the handful of people who walked by exactly when we did.

What happened here? Was this some suicide in protest of the Communist government, and did the guy cut his own throat? Doubtful. Was he killed here and did the murderer get away? Perhaps. Was he the criminal and did the police take him down? Possible, but plausible? There are a dozen other explanations.

In America—and most other Western countries—we would have found out. There would be an investigation. Questions asked and answered. Explanations given. Motives found and understood. They would uncover every detail of this man's life, find his deepest and darkest secrets, and dig up memories even he didn't know he had.

Not in China.

This guy—whoever he was and whatever he did and however he died—wasn't just killed. He was erased. There is no sign of his death, and I suspect that soon there will be no sign of his life. He has been removed from the narrative of Chinese history with maximum efficiency and no delay. Delays mean time and time means observation and observation means questions and questions mean doubt. If there is one thing the government will not allow—not in this location and certainly not on this date—it is doubt. To erase doubt, China must erase the body.

If the Chinese populace ever finds out about this, it will likely be a twisted account. Chinese news will call this man "a foreigner" and "a terrorist." He attacked "the state." He was "a threat." And now he has been eliminated.

Only now do we see the government at work, forcing the people to see a predefined perspective and making them believe a predetermined version of events. In reality, someone was killed in front of the Forbidden City, across the street from Tiananmen Square. In the Chinese alternate universe, it is another beautiful day in the nation's capital, and there is nothing out of the ordinary to worry about or fear. ·

Nearby, a giant portrait of Chairman Mao smiles down on the street. In a very real sense, this is his world, and we're just living in it.

A few days later, as we say goodbye to Chairman Mao and his country, J. J. does us a huge favor. She writes on a napkin in Mandarin: "Please take us to the airport. Terminal 3. Please use the meter." The following morning, we hand that to a cab driver and board a flight for our final stop in Asia.

Chapter 21

May 26, 2014
35°41'48.4"N 139°47'35.6"E
Tokyo, Japan

If a race of alien beings came down from outer space and asked to see humanity's best example of sport, you would not offer up two scantily-clad, vastly overweight men hurling themselves at each other as the paradigm of athletic achievement. You could make a compelling case for soccer or basketball, but certainly not sumo wrestling.

And yet I can hardly think of a better way to spend an afternoon than watching a sumo tournament in Tokyo with my parents, who have flown halfway across the world to join us on this part of our tour. I am sure the novelty wears off at some point (as it did for us after the third hour), but it's a delightful way to spend those three hours, partly because it is quite amazing how big some of these sumo wrestlers are, and also because the ceremony that surrounds each bout is fascinating.

First, a bit about sumo wrestling. Some estimates place sumo's origins approximately 1,500 years ago. The first organized tournament was held around the 1680s as a result of the sport's growing popularity, but the sport existed long before that. Legend has it that it was a way to entertain the gods or perhaps a sport handed down from the gods. The sport itself is incredibly simple. Two guys stand in a ring. The winner is the first to get the other guy off his feet or out of the fifteen-foot ring, called a *dohyo*. Experience certainly helps, but weight helps even more. Sumo wrestlers eat *chankonabe*, a stew of fish, meat, and vegetables, to help them put on weight as

quickly as possible. The largest athlete in human history was a sumo wrestler. Emanuel Yarbrough stood at a height of six feet seven inches, and he
weighed 882 pounds at his heaviest. He also wasn't Japanese—he hailed
from Rahway, New Jersey, a city that has no sumo culture at all (I say that
confidently, having grown up about forty-five minutes south of there. My
high school did not have a sumo team, though in hindsight I wish it had).
In addition to sumo, Yarbrough competed in wrestling, football, mixed
martial arts, and judo, making him one of the most famous sumo wrestlers
outside Japan. He died on December 21, 2015 of a heart attack at the
tender age of fifty-one.

There are six sumo tournaments each year, three of which are in the
Ryogoku in Tokyo, the official sumo hall. Sumo wrestling has been broadcast live on Japanese TV virtually every year since 1953, making it one
of the first sports you could watch live. I imagine watching sumo on live
television would be much like watching American football. There are brief,
spastic moments of euphoric excitement that last perhaps three or four
seconds, followed by a few minutes of downtime. Then more excitement,
then downtime, excitement, downtime, etc. The excitement-to-downtime
ratio leans disproportionately toward the latter half of the equation, and
yet both sports bring in millions of viewers in their respective countries.

By a stroke of luck—if one can call it that—we end up in Japan during
the May tournament. There are six divisions of sumo. The rookie divisions wrestle in the morning; the experienced divisions wrestle in the early
afternoon and evening. Sumo connoisseurs are fully aware of this and will
not bother showing up until later in the day when the well-known sumo
wrestlers compete. We are not sumo connoisseurs.

Eager to witness our first sumo match, we show up early and immediately run headlong into the rituals that surround each sumo tournament. The
elaborate ceremonies that precede every match are completely foreign to us,
yet oddly entertaining. Sumo wrestlers march in together in two rigid lines,
circle the *dohyo* and perform a ritual dance, then regularly throw salt in the
ring in order to purify it from evil spirits. Each wrestler performs a spiritual
dance before a bout, then gets into position and awaits the referee's signal.
After a few more minutes of ceremonies and rituals and traditions, the bout
itself lasts about three seconds. Two very large men hurl themselves at each

other with frightful force. One tends to be larger than the other, the smaller one generally falls back or is pushed out of the ring, and the bout ends as quickly as it began. The referee points his accordion-like fan at one of the sumo wrestlers to declare the winner. Incidentally, sumo is written with the Chinese characters that translate to "mutual bruising," which would make a great name for a heavy metal band.

We settle in to watch two hours and fifty-five minutes of ceremony and five minutes of sumo. We're mostly in an empty square, as we are sumo neophytes and cognoscenti know to arrive later. Having bought cheap seats, we happily move up for a better vantage point, trying to understand the strategy behind such a historic sport. All other things being equal, the difference between good and bad sumo wrestlers is something I cannot possibly divine. Every sumo wrestler looks like he's doing exactly the same thing to every other sumo wrestler, namely throwing himself at the other guy quite recklessly and hoping the gentleman at the other end of the ring weighs a bit less. Yet there are at least eighty-two different winning sumo techniques, all of which look stunningly alike to the uninitiated. After watching a few different levels compete, we conclude we have seen enough of sumo for one round-the-world trip.

My parents share our feelings, which fall at an indeterminable point somewhere between "impressed" and "not impressed."

"It was interesting," my dad says afterward, making it clear that even he is not sure whether he means it in a good or bad way. My mom smiles her big smile. She enjoyed herself simply because she was with us. If asked to describe sumo wrestling after having just seen three hours of it, I'm not quite sure what she would come up with or if it would have any relation to what we just saw.

I can't honestly say that sumo was high on my list of things to do while touring the world—it just happened to work out with our schedule—but Japan itself was always very high on our list. Cassie wanted to see her best friend from second grade, and I was busy shattering all the stereotypes I once held about Eastern culture.

Americans tend to believe that New York City is the most important city on earth and Times Square is the center of the known universe. It's not. In fact, it barely cracks the top ten in metro population, sneaking in behind Beijing but edging out Cairo. Don't get me wrong. A population of nearly nineteen million New Yorkers is an impressive collection of humanity, especially when every single one of them is trying to board the subway at rush hour. But it doesn't compare to Tokyo. Not even close. Tokyo's metro population has nearly thirty-eight million people. New York would be a quaint suburb of Tokyo if the two were placed near each other.

For the sake of humanity, I'm glad the two cities are quite far apart. Take, for example, the aforementioned subway systems. Every day in New York, 5.6 million people cram into twenty-one different subway lines in the most chaotic way possible. There is pushing and shoving, shouting and cursing. An eclectic array of street musicians adds a soundtrack to the cacophony every time the subway doors open, unleashing the human contents inside.

Every day in Tokyo, 8.7 million people cram into thirteen different subway lines in the most orderly way possible. The people waiting to get on the subway queue patiently, allowing other riders to alight before boarding. There is no pushing or shoving, hardly any contact between people, and little need to get angry.

Both systems work—and quite well at that—but they work because they fit the personalities of the people that use them. If you were to mix these two populations of subway riders even slightly, you would likely reignite World War II.

As for Times Square's collection of neon lights, glowing billboards, and oversized advertisements? They seem tame in comparison to just about any street corner in Tokyo. The entire city is lit up in bright, garish colors. What other city offers a combination dinner and cabaret *robot* show in the red light district?

Sadly, we do not buy tickets to the show. It seems an unnecessary expense for a couple on a tight budget, and I decide it's one of those discussions I should not start because I know I will lose. Discretion is the better part of valor.

Before arriving in Tokyo, I had been nervous about seeing my parents again, especially my father. Granted, I saw them only two months ago when we were home, but so much has changed since then, especially my comfort level with diabetes.

When I was home, my dad wanted to see my blood sugar numbers every day, and he would give me constant advice about how to adjust my insulin regimen, despite the fact that no one in the family has diabetes and he has never had reason to research it. Even when we started traveling again, he wanted a daily email with my blood sugar numbers, which I absolutely refused to send more than once a week or so. He tried to manage my diabetes from abroad, telling me to adjust my slow-acting insulin up or down two units based on his calculations. I promptly deleted these emails.

Undoubtedly, he was being a caring father—one I am eternally grateful I have—and I was being a rebellious son. That doesn't mean I despised it any less.

I was worried the process would continue now that we were together and perhaps become even worse. Would he feel compelled to inform me how much insulin I should be taking with each meal? Or how good my blood sugar numbers were? If so, I would feel compelled to explode.

A day before the sumo tournament, we meet them in our hotel. My parents, who have the room next to us, insist we come over to catch up, even though it is obvious to Cassie and me upon arrival that, first, my parents have just woken up from an afternoon nap and are still viciously jet-lagged, and, second, my dad is just about completely naked, save for his underwear. Shame is not something the Liebermanns are capable of experiencing. At least my dad stays under the covers until Cassie and I leave the room.

"How are your numbers?"

"Fine." I hand him my blue notebook where I track my blood sugars, tensing for the fight ahead. He looks them over matter-of-factly before handing the book back. I try not to show my surprise. For weeks, I had been expecting an argument, a lecture, or a suggestion. Instead, he simply nods, and we move on.

A quick shower, and we begin exploring a new city and a new country.

Our first stop is, strangely enough, an intersection. I can't think of any other converging streets in a foreign country that we decided we had to see, but Shibuya Crossing in Tokyo is considered one of the city's most popular sites. It is—and I am trying to muster up as much enthusiasm as possible for this—a five-way intersection. Admittedly, it is a very large five-way intersection, with a few main streets coming together at once, but it is, at its heart, a lopsided crossing of streets, like a pentagon that has shifted a bit to its left.

What is amazing about Shibuya Crossing is the semblance of order that always exists here. Everything—and everyone—follows a neat, timely schedule, controlled by the traffic and pedestrian lights. It reminds me of a school crossing guard guiding a dozen children across the streets while holding cars at bay with a big paddle. Except there is no crossing guard here, and there are thousands upon thousands of children. The second the walking light turns green, the entire intersection fills with a massive crowd of pedestrians walking in every direction, yet never running into one another, as if repelled by one another's electrons.

Near Shibuya Crossing, we stumble upon a sushi-go-round, one of the most efficient meals I have ever experienced. A conveyer belt carries little dishes of sushi around the room. Customers sit around the conveyer belt, choosing which dishes to eat. Cassie sits quietly to my left, munching on our first decent bite of sushi in months, while my mother stares at the entire sushi-go-round apparatus, marveling at its ingenuity while deciding which bit of tuna looks freshest. The price of a meal is determined by the color of the plate. We each eat a few plates, and I spend the meal dividing my attention between picking the cheap colored plates off the conveyor belt and watching my father struggle with his chopsticks.

Eliyahu Samuel Liebermann—a man who has a PhD in aerospace engineering, who built his own airplane, and who started his own engineering firm—cannot, for the life of him, figure out how to use chopsticks. He fumbles with them hopelessly, trying to get the pointy ends to come together without using both of his hands. With each attempt, one chopstick doesn't move while the other wiggles back and forth erratically, never risking contact with the first chopstick. I suspect on some level that chopsticks are too simple for him. When I was in a band in college, our guitarist was unable to play a simple chord progression. He had to complicate it, somehow. I think that's how my dad views chopsticks. Two sticks with no protruding edges that are supposed to come together in some way to grasp food in the middle. He wants to make it more complex than that, despite our repeated instructions.

Never one to admit that there is only one way to solve a problem, he eventually wields his chopsticks like a pair of one-pronged forks, stabbing his food and lifting it to his mouth in a gesture that reminds me of the part in 20,000 *Leagues Under the Sea* wherein Captain Nemo fights off a giant squid by hurling spears at it. The only difference is the scale. My dad hurls a chopstick instead of a spear, and he's aiming for a piece of cephalopod.

Incidentally, my dad despises Japanese food generally and sushi specifically, so we end up eating at more Irish pubs in Japan than we did in Ireland, especially in Tokyo, where foreign food is easy to find. Our sushi-go-round experience is one of our few Japanese meals in Japan.

We spend three days in Tokyo before leaving the very bright lights of the very big city for the countryside. My parents looked at a *National Geographic* tour of Japan for suggestions on what to see, and we simply ripped off the itinerary, adjusting it to our timeframe. From Tokyo we head to Matsumoto, Takayama, and Kanazawa, moving slowly north and west by bus and train. The order of consonants and the cities to which each one belongs escape my parents. As we talk each night about what we have seen, I am never quite sure what or where they're talking about.

"Takamoto was beautiful," my mom says, and I have no idea if she means Takayama or Matsumoto.

"Yes, so was Matsuzawa," my dad responds, creating some hybrid city of Matsumoto and Kanazawa.

"Just like Kanayama."

I don't know if they're referring to the first half of the city or the second, so I politely smile and nod. Maybe Japanese efficiency has caught up with them and they're simply complimenting two cities at once.

We conclude our Japan wanderings in Kyoto. Kyoto is what I expected Tokyo to be, though the confusion is due entirely to my own ignorance and not at all to the city planners who created two diametrically opposed urban environments with names that are anagrams.

Where Tokyo is full of stylish skyscrapers and bright neon lights, Kyoto is replete with ancient Buddhist temples, stunning Japanese architecture, and myriad costumed geishas. We visit too many temples to describe any specific one in great detail, but I do stumble across the grown-up version of something I used to sell.

Back in high school, I spent my senior year working at a store called Natural Wonders. It sold a random collection of science experiments, nature-themed T-shirts, and telescopes. It was a horrible concept for a store. One day, we even registered negative sales, an accomplishment that was only possible because someone made a huge return and we barely sold anything. The only neat thing we sold were ecospheres. They were little enclosed glass baubles that had a few brine shrimp—more commonly known as sea monkeys—swimming around happily in their clear spherical cage. I bought one for my girlfriend. It didn't last long, and here I am referring to both the brine shrimp and the girlfriend.

On the counter near our registers, we sold Zen gardens. The package, which was entirely overpriced at fifteen or twenty dollars, consisted of a small, flat container, some sand, a few stones, and a neat little wooden rake, perfectly sized if a squirrel encountered the sudden urge to do some yardwork. I never quite understood the name at the time, since nothing grows in a Zen garden, and it doesn't seem to inspire a feeling of Zen.

I still don't understand it now, looking at one of the most famous Zen gardens in the world in the temple of Ryoan-ji in northwest Kyoto. A temple has stood on the grounds of Ryoan-ji since the eleventh century. The temple has been torn down and rebuilt a few times—most recently destroyed by fire in 1779—but its most striking and famous feature is the eponymous Zen garden. Historians disagree on when the Zen garden was added to the temple, but estimates put it anywhere between the fifteenth and seventeenth centuries. It is at least a hundred years older than America. Ryoan-ji is considered one of the finest examples of a dry landscape garden.

It is a rectangle of 248 square meters with fifteen rocks in three groups spread out between white gravel. The gravel is meticulously raked every day by the monks. As with any piece of art, there is a wide variety of explanations for what the garden is supposed to represent: islands in a stream, mountains poking out above a layer of clouds, swimming baby tigers, and the list goes on. Sitting on the platform that faces the Zen garden and meditating is supposed to inspire a state of inner peace and concentration.

None of this happens to me while I am staring at the gardens and taking pictures. Part of the problem is the swarm of teenage kids that are careening around the garden, doing very un-Zen things like talking and laughing. But I think most of it is that I'm not properly Zen enough, even though I'm not quite sure what that means. I think this applies to my family as well. Cassie stands by me only because I'm busy taking pictures. My parents take a brief look at the garden and keep moving. And then we are on to the next tourist spot. In fact, the most distinctive memory of the Zen garden is the flashback to my old job.

After a few more days in Kyoto, we part ways with my parents. They have a flight home from Kyoto, while we fly back to Tokyo to catch a flight to San Francisco.

San Francisco may seem a strange place for an American to visit on a trip around the world, but consider this. Our flight from Bangkok, Thailand, to Kathmandu, Nepal, took four hours. A flight from New York to San Francisco takes five hours. It's not exactly a weekend trip. So we take advantage of being on the Pacific Ocean to visit some friends in San Francisco, and Cassie's parents decided to take a week off to meet us there to go romping around wine country in Napa and Sonoma Valleys.

Our flight to San Francisco, to American soil once again, is an easy flight on an easy day. Or at least it should be. We wake up late, have a standard Comfort Inn breakfast in Narita, then head for the airport with plenty of time to spare, which allows us to peruse Japan's bewildering array of Kit-Kat flavors. We buy some Red Bean Kit-Kats, some strawberry cheesecake Kit-Kats, and some pudding Kit-Kats, and head for check-in for Flight 838, only to get a perplexed look from the ticket agent.

"Flight 838?"

"Yes, 838 to San Francisco at 3:50."

"Flight 838 to San Francisco at 3:50?"

"Yes, Flight 838 at 3:50."

This went back and forth for some moments—me naming the flight number, destination, and time in a definitive statement and her repeating the flight number, destination, and time in a question. The intonation in my voice went down at the end of the sentence, and the intonation of her voice went up.

"Flight 838 to San Francisco at 3:50?"

"Yes, 838. San Francisco. 3:50."

"Oh, your flight was cancelled. Please wait in this line for help."

Cancelled? I'm so stunned, I don't even blow up at the lady. A quick check of the departure board confirms this horrible bit of new information. The airline cancelled our flight without giving us any warning. No email, no phone call or text message, no nothing. Thankfully, there are only about six people in front of us in line, so we should be on the next flight to San Francisco, leaving a short time later, right?

After ninety minutes of standing in line, our planned trip to the United States seems to include one more unplanned night in Tokyo. I am ready to blow a gasket and I kindly inform a hapless airline employee that she is a fucking idiot when she tells me I have to use a pay phone to call the reservations line for her company when it is her company's decision to cancel the flight that forces me to make the call in the first place. The Japanese rarely speak loudly, and if I had to guess at their average decibel level, I would say it's somewhere in the sixties. I have surpassed that exponentially, and I wonder if I could apply for the loudest person ever in Japan. In a country renowned for its intelligence, I conclude I am surrounded by idiots, and I try to yell at as many of them as possible, which makes me feel inestimably better while advancing our position not at all.

Cassie, employing a strategy that is completely foreign to me, is nice to a different agent and is allowed to use a company phone for free. Moments later, she informs me that we have the last two seats on the next flight out of Tokyo for San Francisco.

Two things amaze me about this entire debacle. First, that a Twitter message Cassie sent to the airline is far more effective at getting us a new flight than a small army of airline contract workers at Tokyo's Narita International Airport. The airline's social media team responds with a phone number, and, somehow, Cassie does in one five-minute phone call what five airline workers in Tokyo are completely unable to do in an hour and a half.

Second, it seems we will not have a headache-free trip back to the States. Our last flight home involved a five-hour delay, of which three hours were spent sitting on the tarmac at Baltimore-Washington International Airport. And now the airline cancels a flight and hefts upon us a veritably incompetent group of airline employees, in what can best be described as adding insult to injury. Okay, rant over. But be forewarned. Our problems getting back to the United States have not ended.

We land in San Francisco twelve hours before we took off, in one of those strange time-space paradoxes that always happens when you cross the international date line from west to east. Back on American soil, we head straight for a pharmacy and purchase in four minutes what I couldn't find in four countries: a blood sugar monitor that uses the seven hundred blood sugar test strips I have been carrying around.

Then we do what we do best. We head for Napa Valley and drink wine.

A week later, after spending time with friends and family, we board a plane for South America.

Chapter 22

June 12, 2014
13°15′51.4″S 72°26′50.3″W
Machu Picchu, Peru

"No one died at Dead Woman's Pass," our hiking guide, Mike, tells us at dinner, in what I suspect is a tone of voice meant to reassure us. "No one died there. It's called that because it looks like a woman lying down. But *Lying Down Woman's Pass* isn't a good name.

"So . . . Dead Woman's Pass," Mike says, before he helps himself to more rice. He claims he would be thin if they didn't serve such good food on the trail.

We are having our first dinner on the Inca Trail, a four-day trek to Machu Picchu that will take us as high as fourteen thousand feet before we descend into the ancient Incan city. The fact that Dead Woman's Pass has not killed anyone is of little comfort to our exhausted group. We all feel dead, which, as far as we're all concerned at this particular moment, is much the same as *being* dead. It's only day one, and we're wiped.

After my diagnosis, I began to view the Inca Trail as one of the most significant parts of the trip for me. Above all else, it is a big *fuck you* to my diabetes, much as the Great Wall of China was, but on completely different scales. The Great Wall was one night away from civilization and medical care. This is most of a week.

The last time I took on a hike of this magnitude, Cassie and I were in the Himalayas, and the hike almost killed me. Now I am determined to complete this hike to prove to myself—and maybe even to others—that I will not accept any limitations on my life. I control my diabetes. It does not control me.

We meet our hiking group the night before the trek. Fifteen of us, mostly Americans with some Brits and an Aussie tossed in for good measure. Though we are an eclectic mix at first, our guide promises us we will be a family by the end of the hike.

I check my email one last time before calling it a night and see a message from my dad.

"You don't have to be brave. If you don't feel well on the hike, you can stop and turn around. Love, Aba."

It is a nice note, but I delete it almost immediately. I know with absolute certainty that I'm going to do everything it takes to finish the hike, and I'm sure he knows it too. I am willing to put my life at risk once again to make a point.

We set off at five the next morning, settling into our seats for a ninety-minute bus ride to the starting point of the Inca Trail. We grab a small breakfast somewhere along the way—nothing special, but enough to tide us over until we stop for our first snack break. I buy a small bag of coca leaves, the raw material from which cocaine is made, to chew during the hike. Our guide says they help with the altitude.

"Take bits of charcoal, wrap them up in coca leaves, and start chewing." I stuff my bag in my cargo pocket and make it a point to break out the coca on the tough climbs.

At the starting point of the hike, Mike gives us one final pep talk.

"Remember to go slowly. And let us know if you need help." A moment's hesitation. "Packs on!"

Mike pulls me aside. I know what he is about to ask.

"Uh . . . I saw that you are diabetic. Will everything be okay?"

"Yes, I promise you. Everything will be fine. And if the shit hits the fan, Cassie knows exactly what to do."

"Good!"

I think he is reassured that I have a backup plan and relieved that he is not a part of it.

Our group takes a photo by the CAMINO INCA sign that leads to the first checkpoint and the trail. Then we begin. Within minutes the path immediately ascends. Mike had warned us earlier. Today we will climb for ten minutes right at the beginning. Tomorrow we will climb for four hours. Better get used to it now.

In the higher altitude at seven thousand feet, we are all breathing hard after only a few steps. Our porters—called *chasquis* (runners) in Quechua, the native language of Peru—fly by us, effortlessly moving faster while carrying more. We plod along, sucking in every bit of oxygen within vaccuuming range of our lungs.

I push myself because I can. There is no weakness holding me back, no overwhelming thirst slowing me down. Mike prods us all along with cheery phrases like "Easy peasy, lemon squeezy" and "Hola hola, Coca-Cola." These corny idioms become our mottos, and we shout them out as we crest each successive hill, fueling our tired legs with positive energy, which doesn't work quite as well as calories but is a passable substitute until the next snack break.

The first day is the easiest day—not easy, but *easier* than the other days of the hike. We don't climb too much, and we don't walk too much. About seven miles of hiking over eight hours. We all know what awaits us on day two—Dead Woman's Pass, a brutally steep climb up to 14,000 feet, followed by a sharp descent back down to 12,500. By some geographical coincidence, the highest point of Dead Woman's Pass is almost exactly as high as Annapurna Base Camp. At least in theory, the challenge of the climb will be almost exactly the same.

Day three isn't a test of strength. It's a question of endurance, a ten-mile marathon of hiking that will take us twelve hours. We have to climb two mountain passes—neither as high as Dead Woman's Pass but difficult nonetheless—and the rest is Peruvian flat, which is a polite way of saying an endless succession of rolling ups and downs.

Cassie and I move well on the first day, normally within a few steps of each other. Breathing is often difficult, but we catch our breath after a few seconds. It feels great to be here on the Inca Trail, inhaling cold, crisp air as we work our way higher into the Andes.

At dinner that first night, we all begin to get to know one another, swapping stories of where we came from and dreams about where we're going. Chris and Ali—a Scot and an Aussie—are on an extended trip like ours, except they did a lot more skiing. Their next stop is Brazil to see four World Cup matches. After the trek, they take an overnight bus from Peru to Brazil for their first match, and by the time they get off the bus, both England and Australia have been eliminated.

Jim and Cristin—two Americans from New York—are on their delayed honeymoon. They took six weeks off to tour the Pacific Rim. Their next stops will be Buenos Aires, then Sydney. Then there's Dane and Francois— two friends from Missouri who decided it's time for an adventure together for some camaraderie and maybe even a bit of soul searching. And the list goes on. Fifteen different stories from fifteen different people sharing one hike on the Inca Trail.

As I climb into my sleeping bag that first night, a realization hits me. The last time I used this sleeping bag, I was in the first hospital in Nepal. It was during my darkest hours. All sorts of memories come flooding back about the Himalayas trek, the week I was diagnosed, the time in the hospi- tal, and how much Cassie helped me through every minute of those days.

These are painful memories; they will always be painful memories. Now they are still raw, and the emotional scars haven't formed yet.

Cassie is already asleep, but I reach over and place a hand on her arm. She was my rock then, and she is my rock now. I wish I could slide closer and hug her, but she needs her rest. I do too, but sleep suddenly becomes elusive. There isn't a sound in our campsite, and I lie awake in bed, waiting for my eyes to close. Even the simple act of trying to fall asleep reminds me of the hospital in Nepal, when Cassie would leave at night to send emails to my family, and I would be left alone. Once again, I have no way of track- ing the passing time. I slow my respiration and count each breath, trying to figure out how many times I exhale in a minute. Remembering the cramps from the Himalayas, I try to stretch my legs in my sleeping bag.

At least now Cassie is right next to me. And I am feeling great, ener- gized by the physical effort of the hike and the beauty of the surroundings. Easy peasy, lemon squeezy.

The wake-up call comes at 5:30 in the morning. A *chasqui* knocks on our tent—insofar as one can knock on a soft piece of nylon—and whispers, *"Buenos dias.* Coca tea?" The hot drink is a welcome start to the day after a cold night.

Breakfast is a rushed affair with only one cup of coffee, not the neces- sary seven if I'm to function properly any time before 6 a.m. We hike in the pre-dawn light. A short, flat section first, and then we begin the climb to

Dead Woman's Pass. As we begin the push, it occurs to me that I might as well be in Nepal on the Annapurna Base Camp trek. The Inca Trail has the same uneven steps, the same altitude, and, although far from significant, the same color dirt. At least it's not snowing or raining.

We hike under beautiful blue skies, letting the sun warm us even if the air is quite cold.

The air is getting thinner, and we can feel it. We rest often, each time a few moments longer than the one before. I pull out my bag of coca leaves and start chewing, following Mike's instructions. This is the closest I have ever come to doing drugs—chewing on dried leaves and charcoal while hiking in the Andes. I don't know if the coca leaves help, but at least they give me something to do while we climb.

I am tired as we trek, but unlike Nepal, I am not exhausted, and I am not cramping. There is no feeling of weakness, no perpetual thirst, and—thank God—no need to run to the bathroom every hour. If I test my blood sugar and it's low, I eat one of my stash of Snickers bars I have or take one of the glucose gels. With all the trekking and climbing, my blood sugar never gets too high.

It feels awesome to be up here, even invigorating. It is one more step in living the way I intend to, not the way diabetes forces me to. Inevitably, I have to answer all the usual questions as our group sees me taking insulin shots, but it's great to hear the *good for you*'s and the *it's awesome that you're still up here*'s from everyone. On the Inca Trail, we support one another, applauding as everyone reaches the campsite and wishing each other good luck on the next stretch.

The final push to the top of Dead Woman's Pass is the toughest part of the trek. Each step is slow and deliberate. We rest every couple of minutes, sitting on a rock or on the trail for a quick break. Then we keep moving. When we take the last few steps to the top, it is nothing short of empowering. Everyone on the summit—our group and other groups—breaks out into applause and shouts congratulations. At this altitude, it takes me a long time to catch my breath, but that doesn't stop me from smiling at everyone around me. We take pictures at the top, hugging and jumping and sitting and screaming and snapping whatever other photos we can think of.

It takes thirty minutes for all of us to assemble at the top. We are one of the last groups to ascend, and Mike waits until the other groups leave.

We are alone, and it's getting late. We have two more hours of hiking to get down to our campsite for the evening, but Mike holds us up. He leads us to the top of a small mound that offers absolutely no protection from the relentless wind, and he begins whistling. An old Incan spiritual song. Some of us are shivering, but no one cares. There is a feeling of unity and harmony up here. For once, Mike is not telling jokes. He is committed to this moment and this ceremony. So are we.

Mike passes around three small coca leaves (I can't help but notice that he holds them up in the shape of the old Adidas logo). He asks us each to make a wish for *Pachamama*, the Earth Mother, then blow on the leaves three times. He hands each of us an individual leaf and asks us to make a wish for ourselves. Standing up here, with Cassie by my side and my disease under control, I think, *I need not, and I want not.* I am in the middle of nowhere, far away from medical care or even a decent shower, and yet I don't feel that I am lacking in any way.

We place all of our leaves together under a small stack of rocks—one of many small stacks on the surrounding mountainside, each hiding its own set of wishes—and start down toward camp. We walk in silence, savoring the ceremony and the quiet company. We went up the mountain a group and came down a family. Mike was right.

At night, the temperature drops below freezing. Certainly it's cold, but still a far cry from the frigid weather we experienced every night on our Himalayas trek. We huddle together in the blue tarp tent as the *chasquis* serve us dinner. Mike entertains us with ghost stories about the lonely woman—"She haunts a lagoon we will see tomorrow; her husband drowned her before turning himself him in"—and about the poncho man.

"One night I heard a noise—a scraping—on my tent. Like someone pushing against it. I yelled at the person to stop. And it did stop, for a moment. It started again. I opened my tent and looked out. I saw a poncho floating in front of me. A red poncho. But there was no body. The poncho was floating in midair. My assistant saw it too. Then it vanished. A few minutes later, we heard a woman scream like she was being murdered over by the bathroom. She saw the poncho, too."

Mike, always laughing and joking with us on the trail, is absolutely stoic as he steps out of the tent. Some of the girls are absolutely terrified. Even the prospect of going to the bathroom—a two-minute walk away—horrifies them. They start planning their bathroom trips together, just in case they meet the poncho man. They find strength in numbers.

Suddenly we hear a scream outside the tent, and someone—or something?—is pushing frantically against the outside, scraping it with terrible claws. Trying to get in. Or maybe trying to get us out.

The noise and the scraping stop, and we hear Mike's maniacal laughter outside. I start cracking up—the perfect practical joke to follow up a ghost story. Without the need for a tedious vote, the group unanimously hates him this evening. If this were an island, he would be voted off of it in short order, with or without a life raft.

We all go to bed that night having formed new bonds with a group of strangers. On the road, it's that easy to make friends, especially when we're all on one big, brutal hike together.

The third day brings another early wake-up call and two hours of climbing to the second pass. We are refreshed after sleeping, but everyone is walking on tired legs. The trail is taking its toll on our bodies. In the Himalayas, Cassie and I hiked four to five hours a day. Never more than six. Now we are hiking eight to twelve hours. It's exhausting.

We stop at Sayaqmarqa, an archaeological site on the way to Machu Picchu, whose name means *city in the clouds*. It is an apt title, as thick clouds obscure parts of the site.

"Smells like rain," says Edgardo, one of the other guys on our hike. After lunch, he is proven correct. The rain is light at first, but it picks up as we get moving. The flashbacks to our third day in the Himalayas are hard to push aside. Between my undiagnosed diabetes and the miserable weather, that day came very close to breaking my spirit on the hike. Maybe it did a bit. At least it's above freezing. For now.

The rain gets so bad, we are forced to take shelter near the third pass, waiting under a tin roof at a small Ministry of Culture outpost, standing together to stay warm. We may be out of the rain, but the wind seeps through cracks in the walls. Now that we're standing still, our bodies cool down quickly.

After thirty minutes, the rain lets up a bit, and we make a break for it. By the time we reach camp, it is well after dark, but at least the rain has stopped.

We can only afford the luxury of a few hours of sleep on this final night on the trek. The last day of hiking is the earliest wake-up call, so we have as much time as possible in Machu Picchu. We reach the Sun Gate after an hour of hiking. This is supposed to be the first view of the ancient Incan city.

Machu Picchu below you, the rising sun above you.

You're supposed to feel something spiritual here, at peace with the world around you. Mike says it's the perfect place to talk about the history of a marvelous city built in the mountains with an iconic view to take in.

But this morning, the Sun Gate does not live up to its lofty title. The whole area is covered in fog. All we can talk about is the condensation of water at high altitude and the resulting formation of clouds, and since nobody is particularly interested in that topic of conversation, we move on quickly.

We hike along the narrow path down to Machu Picchu, descending without any real sense of how far we are from the Sun Gate or how close we are to the city. Clouds obscure the trail behind us and in front of us, so gauging distance is nearly impossible. Suddenly, there it is. The clouds break, and Machu Picchu is visible.

There are certain places on earth, whether they're landscapes or buildings or scenes, that take your breath away when you see them. In that first instant, they inspire a mixture of awe, wonder, and mystery. There is nothing to do but to stare and try to grasp the beauty of what you are seeing.

Machu Picchu is such a place.

After four days of hiking—you can tell who wasn't used to this kind of living by how fast they reached for their wet naps to clean up at the end of each day—we descend into Machu Picchu.

How—or, for that matter, why—anyone would choose to build a massive stone city high in the Andes Mountains without benefit of forklifts, cranes, or the pneumatic jack is beyond me, when a similar city built at sea level would be both far easier to construct and far more accessible to everyone, including the tourists (though I doubt that profitability and return on investment from future travelers was a major concern during planning). It would be absolutely absurd now to attempt to construct Machu Picchu, given all the red tape and union restrictions, and it must have seemed even more preposterous five hundred years ago, when Pachacutec Inca Yupanqui decided to put his loyal subjects to good use. According to our tour guide, who has read more books on the history of Machu Picchu then I have, the Incas didn't have a tax system. Instead, they paid their taxes through labor, which must have made the city significantly easier to complete. That still doesn't answer the *why* question, but suffice to say it was built at the height of the Incan empire, approximately one hundred years before Spanish conquistadors, armed with new and deadly diseases, wiped out the local population with a dose of smallpox.

Mike leads us around the incredible city, explaining its history and its discovery. Amateur explorer Hiram Bingham discovered the lost city of the Incas in 1911, instantly becoming famous and eventually becoming the sixty-ninth Governor of Connecticut. Bingham's name is all over the area, but he was not the first person to discover Machu Picchu, which would seem to be fairly obvious since a local guide led him to the city. He may not have even been the first Westerner to see it—there's mounting evidence that a German engineer by the name of Augusto Berns mapped the city forty years earlier and tried to raise money to plunder it. At the very least, Bingham is supposed to be the inspiration for Indiana Jones, which is certainly a noteworthy accomplishment in my book.

After a few hours exploring the city, we have a late lunch in Aguas Calientes, the tourist town near Machu Picchu, before most of our group takes the train back to Cuzco. Only a few of us stay in Aguas for one more night. We signed up to hike Huayna Picchu the next morning, the mountain that towers more than a thousand feet above Machu Picchu.

We all take well-deserved showers and relax for a bit, drinking more than a few beers while watching whatever World Cup match happens to be on at whatever bar happens to give us a decent deal on drinks.

We wake up at eight in the morning—it feels like sleeping in—and make our way back to Machu Picchu for the steep one-hour climb up to Huayna Picchu. The view is magnificent, overlooking the city and the mountains. The sky seems endless, stretching effortlessly into the distance, and I admire clouds lazily drifting by in the wind. It is a cool, gorgeous day, and we take our time, enjoying what we have accomplished.

I sit on the edge of the mountain, ignoring Cassie's screams that I am too close to a sheer cliff and that I have zero chance of surviving if I fall. I want to yell back that I won't fall—that I *can't* fall—but that makes far more sense in my head than it would to Cassie. I think it would only reinforce her point.

I stare at Machu Picchu below me and the Andes around me. Breathing in the crisp, thin mountain air, a thought crosses my mind, and I can't help but smile.

I am at peace with my disease.

Chapter 23

July 7, 2014
25°06′42.5″S 65°30′33.2″W
Salta, Argentina

I have often wondered what kind of people plan vacations to places like, say, North Platte, Nebraska, a town of just under twenty-five thousand people that sprouted up a tiny bit southwest of the geographical center of the state. It is a relatively benign three-hour drive north from the geographical center of the United States, located in Lebanon, Kansas, and I find this bit of information nearly irresistible.

I don't know that people do plan vacations to North Platte, but I assume they must, because North Platte has a tourism website. It shows the same five pictures over and over again, one of which is a railyard, which leads me to believe one of the top five things to do in North Platte is to get out of North Platte.

The key marquee on the site touts this rural micropolitan area as one of the premier worldwide destinations to watch the 2017 solar eclipse. This is incredible foresight. As of the time of this writing, that total solar eclipse will happen on August 21, 2017, which is one year, two months and twenty-eight days away. Either that, or there is nothing to do in North Platte between now and then, which, I'm sure the town is loath to admit, is an equally alluring possibility.

I learn the answer to my question—namely, why do people visit such strange places—in San Pedro de Atacama, an even smaller town tucked away in the driest desert in the world in northern Chile. San Pedro de Atacama boasts a population of almost four thousand people, and it looks like it was plucked from the same western movie as North Platte. By some incredible coincidence that I am unable to explain, San Pedro also has an astronomical claim to its fame. Situated at a particularly arid eight thousand feet, San Pedro is one of the best spots in the world to go stargazing, which is why I dragged Cassie with me all the way up here from more normal places like Santiago and Valparaiso. (Convincing her to sit on a twenty-two-hour overnight bus ride to spend a few nights in a budget hostel only to pay thirty dollars each for a good view of the stars certainly qualifies as *dragging* in my book.)

I have only one goal in San Pedro, and that is to take a star tour. A French man and his Chilean wife have set up a telescope farm, which, much to my dismay, is not a place where one grows fresh telescopes out of baby telescope seeds. Instead, twelve telescopes are lined up in neat rows, and we take turns looking through them at exciting cosmic things with equally exciting names, such as globular clusters, binary stars, and lunar landscapes.

Okay, the last one is just the moon, but seeing the moon through a powerful telescope that shows individual craters is far more exhilarating than it sounds. It looks so . . . close. You begin to understand how people in the 1960s looked at the moon, looked at their slide rule, looked at the person next to them, and said, with a confidence that is borderline egomaniacal, "Yeah, we got this."

Unfortunately, *close* is not a word that would accurately describe our next destination. Since there is really nothing to see going north, we have just come from the south, and the Pacific Ocean is west, we decide to head east. We look at a map and pick Salta, Argentina. It seems as good a place to stop as any. The cheapest way to get there is a twenty-hour overnight bus ride, our second overnight bus of the week.

And there is the answer to my question. Occasionally, people must stare at a map of the United States on a cross-country drive, see North Platte staring back at them, and think, *It seems as good a place as any*, which is exactly what we do with Salta. And this must happen often enough to justify the existence and budget of a tourism board that presumably operates the tourism website.

We arrive in Salta late at night. As is often the case upon reaching a new destination, our immediate concern is to find our hostel and locate a place that serves recognizable food. It is this desire to instantly and unequivocally recognize our food and understand what we're eating that draws us to McDonald's for only the third time on our trip. The first was when we had extra euros to spend in Ireland, so I ordered six euros of McDonald's at the Dublin airport before our flight to Hungary. The second was in Hong Kong, where we were exhausted, it was pouring rain, and the large, brightly glowing set of golden arches drew us hypnotically toward it. The third and final time is here in Salta, Argentina.

Of our three international McDonald's excursions, this is perhaps the least justified. There are plenty of other food options, Cassie speaks fluent Spanish, and I speak enough to get by. But it's late enough that we simply don't care. What surprises us is that McDonald's is not fast food here. It's a decent night out.

Back at our hostel, we find ourselves wondering what I suspect many a traveler has wondered in North Platte, Nebraska. What on earth is there to do in this town? To be fair, Salta is significantly bigger than North Platte, with more than twenty times the population. But then again, Detroit has 150 times the population, yet that doesn't make it a tourist destination.

Cassie spots a brochure for a horse ranch an hour outside of town, which is one of the most popular things to do in Salta. It is also probably one of the most popular things to do in North Platte, and this is probably a good place to let this analogy die a peaceful death.

With little else on our agenda, we sign up for an overnight stay, including two days of horseback riding. I am less excited about the horses and more excited about the promised asado lunches—a grill full of beef and sausage and vegetables and lots of wine on the side.

We hitch a cab ride out to the ranch, where we meet our host and, more to the point, our horses. We will return to our host shortly.

There is a reason the mechanical force of an engine is measured in horsepower and not humanpower: horses are immensely, effortlessly, massively powerful. I know this seems intuitively obvious to anyone who was watched a horse race or stood next to a horse. But you cannot truly appreciate that power until you're sitting on top of a horse with little idea of how to control it and even less of an idea of what to do if it decides it's tired of your pathetic attempts at guidance and is ready to strike off on its own in whichever direction and at whatever speed it so desires.

This thought terrifies me, and the thought of it terrifying me terrifies me even more. I have been on a horse exactly once in my life, and that was somewhere in northern New York in a much more controlled environment where the horses are trained not to kick off the riders in the event of any spontaneous disagreements.

Felix, our guide, makes it very clear that no such wisdom has been imparted to these horses. Felix is a true gaucho, having grown up on a horse ranch and herded cattle his whole life. He gives us a few pointers about directing a horse and then, a few seconds later, tells us to follow him. This instruction seems wholly inadequate for the task ahead, like someone telling you how to guide a rocket by pointing you at the ignition and waving goodbye, but it will have to suffice.

Thankfully, the horse seems to know more than I do, which works out well for both of us.

As we near the end of our first outing, Felix looks at us and asks, "Do you want to gallop?"

For someone who loves the idea of going fast and liberally ignores speed limits, this question is a no-brainer, even if I don't have the slightest idea of how to get the horse to go fast or, at some point, to get it to go slow again. The latter seems like a less immediate, but no less important, problem. The notable absence of a brake pedal is worrisome.

To allay my growing concern about my imminent demise, Felix gallops with me the first time, holding the reins of my horse. Then he tells me to go again. Alone.

There have been a few times in my life where I have thought, *I might die in the next few moments if this doesn't go well*. This isn't one of those times. But it briefly crosses my mind that this may not be the best idea. A diabetic amateur rider on a galloping horse seems a recipe for disaster. I'm not sure how the diabetes changes things, but it certainly can't help.

Felix tells me to give the horse a bit of a kick with my heels and make a clicking sound. The horse, reacting instantly, breaks into a gallop.

A galloping horse can move at about thirty miles an hour. To put that in perspective, I have driven three times that fast, flown my own airplane six times as fast, and flown commercially twenty times as fast. In other words, in the grand scheme of things, it's not all that remarkable to gallop on a horse.

Yet the sensation is unlike any other I have ever experienced. The sense of speed is exhilarating. I won't use any trite clichés like *the wind was blowing through my hair* (it is) or *we were moving like a bat out of hell* (we are), but I am so excited by the sensation of galloping on a horse that I instantly smile the sort of smile that can only be described a shit-eating grin. And I am absolutely okay with that.

Felix snaps a picture of me as I go by. It's an absolute mess. It's out of focus, blurry, and looks like his horse was at a full gallop as he took the photo, yet the shit-eating grin is plainly obvious.

That picture still makes me smile every time I look at it.

I am crouched low over the horse, holding the reins tight, trying to keep my nether regions from smashing into the saddle in ways that will permanently limit my ability to have children, and I have a smile from ear to ear. I didn't think riding a horse would be one of my favorite experiences of the entire trip, but it absolutely is.

Back at the ranch, we sit down with our host for lunch. To say that Enrique is rough around the edges would be an understatement. He is the guy who roughed up the edges. He introduces himself with, "I am Enrique. My English is shit." I like him instantly. He is blunt, offensive, and honest, in much the same way that he is hilarious, warm, and genuine.

"*No hay sexa en la mesa,*" he yells at me when I put my arm around Cassie at lunch. There is no sex on the table. Then he breaks into a cackling laughter and refills everyone's wine.

Enrique has grilled every meat available within a two-hundred-mile radius, which is mostly a dozen different cuts of Argentinian beef, with a chicken breast thrown in for good measure only because Cassie prefers not to eat red meat. He speaks disparagingly of chicken, and when he says *pollo* in Spanish with an Argentinian accent that makes it sound like *po-jo,* the *j* in particular is dripping with contempt, as if the chicken breast has profaned his grill by taking up room that could have been used for yet more beef.

He has also grilled an assortment of peppers and tomatoes, and whatever he couldn't grill, he pickled.

"I learned English in Texas. I worked on a horse ranch there when I was young. It was awful. The cowboys called me Mexican all the time."

He searches for the word. "Racism."

"A cowboy is a gay gaucho," he spits as an afterthought.

We have another ride after lunch. Then we enjoy a late, lazy dinner with Enrique and call it a night. In the morning, I decide to do something I've done only a few times on this trip. I shave.

As a general rule, I hate shaving, though I have done it almost every single day of my adult life. There is nothing enjoyable about it, but it has been a professional requirement ever since I started working. Liberated from this never-ending burden to remove my facial hair, I limited my shaving to once every two weeks or so on our trip. I always last about eight days before it starts feeling like fire ants are mauling my face. That's how I know it's time to shave.

The moment Enrique sees me clean-shaven, he starts calling me "Top Model." At first, I think he'll only do this for a few minutes. But he keeps it up throughout the day.

"*Buenos dias*, Top Model!"

"*Como estas*, Top Model!"

"*Salud*, Top Model!"

Apparently, the idea of being clean-shaven on a horse ranch is a bit of a novelty. Enrique himself sports a pepper-gray goatee.

In return, I start calling Enrique "*Mi Amor.*"

We keep the nicknames going through lunch and as we say our good-byes.

"I will return, *Mi Amor.*"

"I hope so, Top Model."

It's a promise I intend to keep.

Two days later, we catch our final overnight bus of our trip—eighteen hours from Salta to Mendoza, where we do our best to drink all the wine in Argentina's best known wine region. We mount a noble effort, but are ultimately unsuccessful, though not for lack of trying.

We find ourselves in Argentina during the semifinals and finals of the World Cup. I will not go into great detail about what it's like to watch World Cup elimination games in the country that's playing in those games. Suffice to say there is nothing that even comes close in the United States. In the largest sporting event of the year—the Superbowl—two cities go wild for a game that's being played in a third city that doesn't care about the game.

In the World Cup, entire countries celebrate, cheer, and go crazy together. When Argentina won the semifinals against the Netherlands, we could hear the celebrations from our sixth-floor hotel room, and they went on all night. Even after the finals, which Argentina lost to Germany, there was about an hour of silence before the country collectively realized it had just finished second in the world.

The celebrations began anew.

The day after the World Cup finals, we make our way back to Santiago to catch a flight home. Or at least we try to. Cassie's brother is getting married on Saturday, and it's fairly critical that we be there.

Mendoza is a short bus ride away from Santiago, so we book tickets for the six-hour ride.

When we arrive at the bus station, my suspicions from Japan are confirmed. We will never have an easy trip home. Our flight from Santiago to Philadelphia is still on time—at least it should be since it's not for another two days. But our bus from Mendoza to Santiago, without which our flight from Santiago to Philadelphia does us absolutely no good, is cancelled. A snowstorm in the Andes has closed down the road and made the mountain pass impassable.

In fact, every bus that left before our bus made it through the pass. The 8:30 and 9:30 buses are well on their way to Santiago. But the 10:30 is stuck in Mendoza, on the eastern side of the pass, while our destination is on the western side. Naturally, the pass will open again when the weather warms and the snow melts, but with the worst of the blizzard still to hit the Andes, it won't open in the two days that we have before our flight.

Once again, our seemingly simple plans to get back to the US have run into an imaginary yet solid wall that I can't help thinking someone intentionally planted there.

We have a few options, but none of them are easy and even fewer are cheap. Unfortunately, waiting for another bus is not one of these options, which means the money spent on bus tickets is probably lost to us forever, if my understanding of Argentine business practices and return policies is correct.

We can try to fly to Santiago, which seems like a great option, except the only airline that flies direct abuses the monopoly and extorts passengers to the tune of $650 for a one-hour flight that should cost $200 at most.

One of Argentina's main airlines stopped flying the direct route a couple of months ago. If we want to fly with that airline, we have to pay just as much money as the direct flight and go 615 miles east so we can end up 90 miles west. I like flying, but not that much.

We end up rerouting our Chile-Philadelphia flight through Buenos Aires instead of Santiago. We will get in a few hours later, but still within plenty of time for the wedding. Our path now takes us from Buenos Aires to Toronto to Philadelphia.

Now we only need to get to Buenos Aires. A bus from Mendoza takes some twenty hours, so that's almost immediately out of the question. Buses that long are almost always overnight, which doesn't give us enough of a margin of error in case something goes wrong again, which it seems to do every time we try to get back on American soil.

Our best bet is to fly, which is easy enough. The Argentine airline offers a whole bunch of daily hops between the two cities. We hop online, place our reservations, and promptly run into the strangest problem I have ever encountered in an online transaction. The company website acknowledges that we have a reservation, tells us we have to pay, and then won't let us pay. We try three different credit cards, and the airline's website keeps telling us to try later, while simultaneously telling us we only have an hour to pay before the reservations are thrown out.

We close out of the window, hoping to try again, but our confirmation email contains no link or mention of how to pay. It only tells us we have yet to pay without telling us how to accomplish this task that's at the core of every business transaction in the history of mankind. Whether buying a car or bartering for a log canoe, one person sells something and another person buys it with some form of payment. Apparently, the airline's business development unit missed this basic lesson when designing their reservations website. We have a product we want to buy and a set price that we have agreed to, but no means of offering compensation in return.

We keep ending up on the same itinerary page that taunts us mercilessly with its ceaseless countdown until our reservation expires without providing us a means to stop the countdown. Someone at the airline is playing a cruel joke on us.

Cassie is very close to tears of frustration. I run down to the front desk to get help from the receptionist, who calls the airline immediately. He, too, is just as perplexed as us, especially when the woman who answers the phone at the airline's corporate phone number insists that the website is working fine, notwithstanding all of the growing evidence to the contrary.

She acknowledges our problem, understands our problem, even tries to solve our problem for a brief moment, then denies that there ever was a problem and hangs up. I am no expert in Spanish, but I know enough to understand that there is a large, unbridgeable gap between making progress and whatever it is that we're doing right now.

I end up walking to the office in person to pay for the tickets, trying to explain to them that their website seems to have been designed by flailing madmen who either don't understand the need for satisfactory payment or have chosen to forgo it entirely. The clerk shrugs, takes my credit card, and hands me our tickets.

We spend one more night in Mendoza before catching a flight to Buenos Aires, where we have a short day to explore. The Buenos Aires metropolis has thirteen million people, which means we spend less time here per capita than in any other city we have visited.

But we will be back.

Chapter 24

July 19, 2014
40°36'21.3"N 75°32'06.6"W
Allentown, Pennsylvania

I wake up in the United States. This is a minor surprise, since I'm not
supposed to be here yet. It is even more of a surprise since I have no
memory of swapping South America for North America.

I remember absolutely nothing about the flight from Buenos Aires
to Philadelphia. There was a layover in Canada, but I don't remember
that either. I only know there must have been one because my tickets
insist on it. I think I was shell-shocked—emotionally numb and mentally switched off as we made our way back home.

When we started traveling, it was almost impossible to believe
that our first month had passed. Then our second month. As we said
goodbye to Europe, it was unreal to us that we had already knocked
off one continent. Even if we savored every moment of every day,
time still flew by in large blocks of weeks and months.

To wake up one morning and discover we are on a flight home
is difficult to believe. So difficult, in fact, that I don't remember the
flight home.

Our trip isn't over yet. We have three more weeks planned in
Buenos Aires and southern Argentina to explore Patagonia, but I suspect these three weeks will have a far different feel to them. In a
sense, they are not part of our incredible journey. They are a regular
vacation before we go back to work, and I can't shake that thought
from my mind.

It is without a doubt financially idiotic to fly home for a wedding, then fly back to the same place we left to resume the last little bit of our trip. Yet, for once, we simply don't care about the finances. We have budgeted our entire trip, and we saved this last bit to make sure we could finish what we started. Six months ago, diabetes forced me to take a month away from our travels. I promised Cassie that I would not give up any more of the trip. We will finish this trip on our terms.

Two days after returning home, we are at Cassie's brother's wedding. The wedding is a blast, and I get to wear the suit I had custom-tailored for dirt cheap in Hoi An, Vietnam. The bride and groom put cards all over the tables that say "Instagram! #AlainaAndAndy." I am very tempted to log on and send out "Upload your amateur porn pics! #AlainaAndAndy."

From the wedding, we head straight for the beach for Cassie's family vacation at the Jersey Shore.

Given how close our trip is to officially being over, Cassie and I both decide to take advantage of the time at home and begin the job hunt. A corporate headhunter we befriended in Seville in October sets me up with an interview at a public relations firm in New York City. I steal a day away from the beach and drive into the city for the interview.

The questions naturally turn to why there is a one-year gap on my resume, which quickly becomes a fun conversation about our trip. At the end of the interview, I am given a proofreading quiz. My interviewer looks over my editing skills briefly, then gives me homework. I haven't had homework in nearly a decade, so the idea of doing serious work while I'm not at work doesn't appeal to me, but this means the interview went well, so I oblige.

The interviewer tells me to put together a marketing plan for the Food Bank of New York City's announcement of a new program. I shake his hand, say thank you, and make my way to the car, pondering what is now the most important question I have to answer.

What the hell is a marketing plan?

I have read countless press releases and been the target of marketing plans aimed at drumming up media attention, but I've never written a plan myself. I also, as a matter of habit, delete press releases the moment they arrive, with the unfortunate consequence that I have read very few of them.

For the next two days, I hunker down in the ice cream and coffee shop near our rented apartment at the beach. The coffee shop has Internet and, more to the point, coffee. My first mission is to figure out what goes into a marketing plan, which takes most of the first day. The second day is devoted to writing one of my own.

In order not to overstay my welcome at the shop, I keep ordering coffee every hour or so. I drink the first three coffees, leisurely sip the fourth, then stop drinking them altogether. I order the coffee, let it sit on my table until it's achieved a completely unpalatable degree of lukewarmth, take one sip, make a horribly disgusted face, and order another coffee. By the third time I do this, the nice young girl in the purple shirt operating the cash register thinks I am patently insane, wondering why I persist in ordering coffees that I have no intention of drinking.

Cassie comes in, sees my thirty-dollar bill, and asks, "How many coffees did you drink?"

"Three."

I send in the marketing plan on a Thursday morning. Over the weekend, Cassie submits an application to a charter school in Harlem. The school emails Cassie the following Sunday to ask her to come in for an interview.

Less than twenty-four hours later, an email pops into my inbox.

Monday, July 28, 2014 at 7:43 p.m.
Michael Smith
To: Oren Liebermann
Subject: RE: Checking in

Hi, Oren,

Having reviewed your writing sample, we're pleased to invite you back for a second-round interview to meet with Jason Gelnovatch and some other members of the team. Are you available, by any chance, this Thursday at either 10 a.m. or 4 p.m.? Just as a heads up for your scheduling, these interviews often take a few hours.

Looking forward to it,
Michael

I am supposed to be elated. I have another interview with a public relations firm in New York City. I am one successful afternoon away from a job offer, and I have barely started job hunting. In ways that I cannot quite explain, life seems to be falling back in order.

Instead, I feel numb. The interview came faster than I expected, which leaves us with no choice. I have to call off the rest of the trip.

For the second time this year, I have forced us away from what we love most. I have taken us off the road. The reasons are entirely different—the first time was for my diabetes; the second is for a job—but the end result is the same. Because of me, we are not traveling. Because of me, we will put our passports away again.

Because of me.

We planned to travel for a year. I have cut that down twice now. We lost a month in the middle of the trip and now we're losing our final month. I have robbed us of the ability to finish the trip on our terms.

Cassie and I unpack our backpacks for the final time and start figuring out where we'll live and how we'll buy a car and all sorts of tasks we haven't thought about in a year.

I schedule a follow-up doctor's appointment for one of the most important tests used in long-term treatment of diabetes, called HBA1C. In technical terms, HBA1C is glycated hemoglobin. It develops when hemoglobin, a protein that carries oxygen throughout the body, joins with glucose. Because these red blood cells renew every three months, measuring HBA1C is a way of measuring your average blood sugar over the last twelve weeks. In non-technical terms, your HBA1C needs to be between 5 and 7. A normal person's HBA1C is 5.6 or lower.

After I was diagnosed in late February, my HBA1C was 12.1. That is well above the dangerous mark. An HBA1C of that level will guarantee severe long-term complications from diabetes, and those complications will come quickly and irreversibly.

So it is with a fair amount of trepidation that I march myself back into the doctor's office to find out how I've been doing in the six months since my diagnosis. I have been strict with recording everything I eat, my blood sugars, and how much insulin I take with each meal. If, having done all this, my HBA1C is still dangerously high, I don't know what more I can do. Then my disease will truly have broken me.

Unfortunately, the HBA1C is not an instant test, at least not in my doctor's office. A nurse draws blood, sends off the sample, and the results come back two or three days later.

When I call in to find out the results, I am nervous. Very nervous. More so than any one individual blood sugar test, the HBA1C is a scorecard to see if you're winning or losing. There are degrees of success here, but anything above 7 is some degree of failure.

"Hi, I'm calling to find out my hemoglobin."

"Your name?"

We go through the rigamarole of them confirming that I am who I say I am and that they are really, truly, honestly allowed to give me medical information about myself.

"You wanted your hemoglobin?"

"Yes."

"Let me see. Your hemoglobin is 12.5."

I am in absolute shock. For weeks, I had no idea what I was doing to my body and my HBA1C was a 12.1. Now, after learning about diabetes and doing everything I could to protect myself, my HBA1C has only gone up.

"That's my A1C? My A1C is 12.5?"

"Oh no, that's your hemoglobin. Let me check your A1C." Relief washes over me. I have just learned in a way that ensures I will never forget that there is a difference between hemoglobin and A1C.

"Your HBA1C is 5.6."

I am beyond elated. Words like *thrilled* and *excited* and *ecstatic* don't quite cover it.

Above all else, I am healthy.

It may seem an insignificant number, especially over the course of the rest of my life with diabetes. But it marks a healthy new beginning for me, and it sets the bar high. We go out to my favorite steak restaurant to celebrate. Cassie gives us one more reason to rejoice. The charter school where she interviewed offered her the job after she gave a demo lesson. It's great news, even if the public relations firm doesn't offer me a job.

The good news is enough to blunt the disappointment of us calling off the last bit of our trip. But it's still lingering there. I don't need to ask Cassie to know that she feels the same. We'll have to visit Argentina again one day to see all that we haven't seen.

One day.

I head into New York City to hang out with some friends and share the news that we'll be hanging out a lot more in the near future. It feels great to sit with friends whom I haven't seen in so long, and I am able to forget for now that our trip ended unexpectedly, earlier than it was supposed to.

As I'm sitting with my friends, my phone starts beeping. Cassie has sent me a few messages.

Her school wants her to start on the following Monday. She tells them that's not quite possible because we aren't set up in any way to start working yet. She promises we will have all that set up in a week, and she would start the following Monday.

The last message makes me smile.

"I booked tickets to Iceland. We leave on Monday."

Chapter 25

August 6, 2014
64°08′50.0″N 21°57′01.6″W
Reykjavik, Iceland

Iceland is a land of indescribable beauty, and it's not because I don't know the words to describe it. It's because you can't pronounce anything in this entire country. Reykjavik is the capital, Eyjafjallajökull is their famous volcano, and *hafragrautur* is their word for something as simple as oatmeal. They apparently harbor a disdain bordering on outright hatred for vowels. With names that sound like an angry Viking threw a Scrabble board against the wall and picked the highest scoring words, asking someone for directions is tantamount to vehicular suicide.

"How do I get to kwfkkwakak?"

"Go four kilometers down the road to kakwelllbd. Turn left when you see the kwellewakwk. Slow down at the bnndnnwielll. When you see the fifth vttvvwaaw, you have arrived." Now I understand why Moses wandered forty years in the desert. He asked an Icelander for directions.

Thankfully, we have a very simple plan that basically guarantees that we won't get lost: stick to one road and don't stray. Of course, that doesn't stop me from putting us on the right road in the wrong direction, but that mistake becomes apparent quickly enough, and after a few sincere apologies to Cassie, we're headed the right way. Once again, we are heading east, this time along Iceland's Ring Road, a two-lane road that follows the circumference of the entire island.

We tossed together a plan for Iceland in a couple of days, scouring a few websites, jotting down a few notes, and heading for the airport. I have never been so excited for a flight. I could barely sit still during boarding, which annoyed Cassie to no end. In the airport, I held out my arm repeatedly to escort her to the gate as if we were both going to the junior prom, except I wasn't nearly this excited for the prom. This is bigger than a night of angst-filled dancing to modern pop music that transitions to overmodulated oldies halfway through the evening. This marks the end of our year abroad, and we are thrilled to finish it here, on our terms.

I am caught up in the excitement of traveling again, of experiencing the world, of meeting people. Less than a week ago, it looked like our trip was over. Cassie had to start her job, and I had to find my own. For a moment—a quick blip of a few days—we put that all on hold. The five-to-nine determined the nine-to-five, not the other way around as it had been for so many years. We will soon be busy making a living, but we will never again forget to make a life.

There is no bittersweet ending here. We have nothing to be upset about. When we got back on the road for this last week, many of our friends—I would even go so far as to say most of our friends—thought we were crazy. They were more than happy to voice their opinions that we had the rest of our lives to travel and that we should now stay home and focus on what they consider to be real life. They failed to realize that, for us, this is real life. We live for travel. All of the other daily tedium—work, taxes, bills, insurance—are simply a means to an end. We go through those motions so we can travel. Isn't that what's real?

We land in Reykjavik early in the morning and head straight for the thermal pools, as tired as we were on our first day in Rome. The time change doesn't favor our schedule, but we are veterans at overcoming jet lag now. We soak in the impossibly blue water, melting in the natural heat. When we step out, the cold air bites our skin and reminds us that we are far closer to the Arctic Circle than the equator. It is summer in the States, with temperatures creeping toward ninety degrees. They haven't discovered summer here. A warm day is sixty degrees. A cold day would send my nuts into my throat looking for warmth.

The following morning, we set out from Reykjavik under gray skies and intermittent rain, which changes to blue skies and a light wind, which becomes steady showers, all in five minutes. What doesn't change is the breathtaking landscape. The island looks like a different planet, more akin to the frozen surface of Saturn's moon Titan than anything terrestrial. The dips and hills resemble thousands of craters, and the volcanic surface reminds me of the moon (which I haven't visited yet, but it's on the list). We marvel at this fantastic display of nature, often stopping by the side of the road for pictures or simply to stare in silence at yet another incredible phenomenon crafted by the relentless forces of wind and ice and tectonic turbulence.

This windswept slab of volcanic rock, stuck way up near the North Pole, isn't exactly overflowing with flora—most of the plants here look like stunted shrubs—but the views are incredible as we venture into the land of Thor and Leif Erikson. We stare at the violent north Atlantic on one side, and the country's famous volcanoes, glaciers, and waterfalls on the other. In many ways, Iceland reminds me of Hawaii. I've never been to Hawaii, but one is a hot volcanic island and the other is a cold volcanic island, so the analogy is probably apt.

Near a Viking museum with a replica longship, a giant Viking sword, at least twenty feet tall, sticks out of the ground in the middle of a traffic circle. Most cultures would shy away from an ancestral history of raping and pillaging. Not Icelanders. They celebrate their Viking heritage by eating small bits of rotten shark and washing them down with Brennivin, a potato liquor flavored with caraway. I am upset when I miss a chance to try this liquor, even as my liver celebrates its pardon from this potable punishment.

We make our way along the southern coast of Iceland, never more than a few miles from the ocean. Signs for natural phenomena pop up every couple of minutes along the road. We see markers for the countless waterfalls—for Seljalandsfoss and Skogarfoss and Gullfoss and all sorts of other fosses. Or the thermal geysers at a place cleverly called Geysir. There is no end to the natural beauty here, and we drive long stretches quietly as we admire the world around us. We find no need to talk here, no need to interject the white noise of our voices. I know Cassie is marveling at what she sees, and she knows I'm doing the same.

The beauty of Iceland speaks to us in ways that do not require a response. We hear nature's words and stories in silence, listening to the ambient noise for the marvelous symphony it is. We dare not disrupt the natural music with anything as simplistic and unworthy as the waveform static of our vocal cords, just as we dare not interrupt Bach's Fugue in D Minor with Kesha's "We R Who We R."

We let the natural wonder sweep over us, often holding hands to add a physical connection to the emotional and spiritual bond we already share. This journey has brought Cassie and me closer than ever before, and we don't need words to express that when our mutual silence during some of the most amazing and impressive moments of our trip says it so much better.

Instead, we save our breath for venting about Iceland's ridiculous prices. A burger that should cost eight dollars sets us back twenty-four. A cup of coffee is upward of nine dollars, and a beer is about twelve dollars. We had traded three weeks of Argentina for five days of Iceland, but the former is so cheap and the latter so expensive that the price works out to be the same. The only inexpensive meal we can find is a three-dollar hot dog in downtown Reykjavik at the country's most popular restaurant. In true Icelandic fashion, the hot dog stand is called Baejarins Beztu Pylsur.

I get that they have to import just about everything they eat, but nearly all of the electricity here comes from renewable thermal energy, so the cost of overhead should theoretically be low. Yet a single bunk in a dorm room still goes for seventy dollars a night, which makes Iceland the most expensive place we've been to by far. I'm glad we're here at the end of the trip and not the beginning. Iceland would've bankrupted us in a week.

Once again, we are heading east, away from home. Away from our family and friends toward another unknown. In our circumnavigation of the globe, we have passed our starting point, and we have started another circle. The end of one journey is the beginning of another.

In five days, we make it as far as Vik, about 110 miles from the capital, where we explore the volcanic black sand beaches at the southernmost point in Iceland. Most people would consider this weather absolutely awful. The wind never stops howling, the precipitation in its various forms never stops spitting, and it's always some degree of cold. We love it. We bundle up in our waterproof jackets that are no longer waterproof, our weather-resistant pants that let through every drop of rain, and our hiking shoes with the long-forgotten treads, and walk straight onto the frigid Iceland beaches, happy to be here.

In this sublime moment.

This perfect ending.

Flocks of puffins—birds resembling parrots with colorful faces and beaks—fill the air around us, diving down into the ocean to grab a mouthful of fish, and we stare at these birds and their great, lazy circles for as long as we can hold out against the cold. Then we warm up with hot coffee that burns our mouths and our wallets while the car heater runs at full blast to thaw out our frozen feet. When we're ready, we step out again.

We explore little caves and grottoes between the volcanic boulders that litter the beaches and oceanside cliffs. I take so many pictures that I drain one camera battery after another. In a sense, we feel unstoppable. We set out to explore the world for a year—to learn about places and people and food and cultures—and we have succeeded, despite setbacks and challenges. Travel tested us in ways we could never have anticipated, and I'd like to think we passed these real life exams. The demands of life on the road either push a couple together or drive them apart—there is no middle ground. We have been brought together.

In so many ways, Iceland is an explorer's paradise (except for the aforementioned outrageous prices). Mother Nature concentrated some of her best offerings on one tiny island, and we try to see as much as possible. In summer—and it is summer here, at least in terms of time of year if not in temperature—the sun barely sets. We enjoy twenty hours of sunlight a day. Because we go to bed at 10:00 p.m. and wake up at 7:00 a.m., we never see darkness. Although it throws off our internal clocks, the constant light gives us as much time to drive and walk and see as we want. Our days, and our lives, are brighter than they were one year ago. If we came back in six months, we would experience the opposite—twenty hours of darkness.

While riding small Icelandic horses one afternoon—don't you dare call them ponies or you will piss off the entire country, regardless of how much these quadrupedal mammals look like miniature versions of *equus ferus caballus*—we ask our guide how they deal with the winters here.

"In winter, we sleep all the time. In summer, we never sleep," he says. I didn't know you could trade six months of sleep for six months of awake, but apparently they've figured out a way.

We go to bed each night tired but fulfilled, exhausted but overjoyed. For all we have seen on our trip, we have the privilege of sneaking in a bit more right at the end.

There have been so many endings on this trip. The end of Europe. The end of Africa. The end of my life without diabetes. But for each ending, there is a new beginning. The beginning of Southeast Asia. The beginning of the Inca Trail.

The cycle never ends.

It keeps going.

As long as you want it to keep going.

On the flight home—Icelandair 615 from Kelflavik to JFK—I put on *The Secret Life of Walter Mitty*. It seems appropriate; it is about a daydreamer who travels the world when things get bad at work. Although my professional life was going exceedingly well when we left forty-seven weeks ago, the first part of the description seems incredibly fitting. I have been guilty of daydreaming my whole life, as evidenced by twelve years of lackluster report cards in grade school and only slightly less lackluster grades in college. Now I am guilty of traveling too.

I thought I would spend most of the flight catching up on cinema, but I find myself staring out the window at the world passing by below us. We are mostly above water, but ninety minutes in we fly over what I'm pretty sure is Greenland, mostly because it isn't at all green. The mountains and icebergs of a country far more remote and desolate than any place we have ever been—except maybe West Virginia—remind us that we have so much left to explore and so many places left to see. I snap a few pictures of the landscape thirty thousand feet below, knowing full well they will be some of the last pictures of this trip.

As I stare out at a distant layer of stratus clouds (and the Icelandair logo on the wingtip of the 757 invading the sanctity of my window view), I have to hold back a few tears. Not tears of sadness that the journey is over. Tears of joy, as full of happiness as the tears I cried on February 19 when my blood sugar finally came back normal and I knew I was on my way home. I feel joy for everything we have seen and done. Everyone we have met. Everywhere we have been. And, perhaps most importantly, everywhere we will go.

Cassie and I sit in the last row—her in the aisle, me by the window. Our preferred seats. The lone seat between us is empty. Only my camera, with my 55–250 mm zoom lens, sits on the pillow that neither of us is using. The tray table is open, the cup that held the official last glass of wine of the trip already removed.

On the thirty-third and final flight of our trip, I am thankful to have the window seat in the last row. I will be the last one off this plane, the last one to step foot on American soil. I will be the last one home, which means I will be the last one still traveling.

My flight—my journey—will last just a few seconds longer than everyone else's. In that brief time, I will be on the road a little bit longer. An extra moment to call myself a nomad, a wanderer, and to think of this trip in the present tense.

Home is both ahead of us and behind us. Our family, our friends, are in front of us. The physical place that we both refer to when we use the term *home* is a short drive from JFK airport, where we will arrive in about three hours as I write this from seat 41A. We have already talked about possible places to live and renting a car and finding work. We will fall back into a normal routine faster than we'd like to admit, I suspect. We will find a one-bedroom apartment, argue over what we can afford, and then we will move in. We will, by most accounts, be home.

But home is also behind us. The stimulus of movement. The excitement of a different city. The trains and buses that became our bedrooms and living rooms. The people we met who turned into our friends and family. We are accustomed to life on the road, used to eating rice and eggs or ordering what passes for pizza or tacos in many parts of the world. That is where we are most comfortable. That is where we are home. For us, *home* is a verb.

We have left too many lands undiscovered and too many oceans unexplored. For everything we have seen and all the cultures we have learned about, we know there are many more to discover in the world's great vastness that we simply know as being "out there." We will go "there" one day. That I know.

We touch down at JFK early in the evening and taxi to our gate. In a few moments, I will trade the interior of an airplane for the interior of John F. Kennedy International Airport's International Arrivals Terminal. Our year abroad will come to an end. I don't know that I'm ready to make that transition, reversing the change we made last September. But, at least for now, I have no choice.

The captain turns off the "fasten seat belts" sign and every passenger rushes to get their bags and get off the plane. Every passenger but me. I am in no hurry, and I see no reason to rush. The calmness of an airplane in flight morphs into the chaos of an airplane at the gate, but I move without haste, deliberately trying to remember every detail of these moments, which will be the last of our trip.

Slowly at first, then all at once, passengers step out of the cabin and onto the gangway and into the airport. It will be my turn in a few seconds. I grab my camera bag and make my way to the door, passing the handful of flight attendants remaining on board. They will clean up the cabin and prepare it for the next flight, as they have done countless times before. For them, and for many of the passengers, this flight was nothing special. It was an ordinary means of transportation from point A to point B. Not for me. Not for us.

As I take one last look at the airplane before heading into the terminal, to customs, to baggage claim, to our taxi, and to home, I realize something.

The journey isn't over.

It's just beginning.

Epilogue

April 28, 2015
28°04'30.6"N 34°30'38.5"E
Gulf of Aqaba

There is no good reason for me to be on this flight. There are, however, quite a number of reasons for me *not* to be on this flight, all of which I knew in advance and none of which I paid attention to. Like many journalists chasing a story, I kept pushing and pushing until I got exactly what I asked for: a free trip to Kathmandu.

A massive 7.8 earthquake had rocked the Nepali capital. The number of dead was in the hundreds and climbing fast. Buildings in Kathmandu had either collapsed or were teetering dangerously close to collapse. Streets were covered in rubble. There was no way of knowing how many people were trapped in the wreckage . . . and still alive.

Nepal was suddenly the biggest story in the world. Foreign aid flooded in. Or at least it tried to. The earthquake had damaged Kathmandu's single runway, making it impossible for planes over a certain size to land.

Israel had a 747 loaded with personnel ready to go, along with a few C-130s full of medical supplies and a field hospital. I had begged the Prime Minister's Office, the Foreign Ministry, Israel's military aka the Israel Defence Forces (IDF), and a few politicians for a seat on that flight. We had to wait an extra twenty-four hours at Tel Aviv's Ben Gurion Airport until we were sure the Kathmandu runway was in suitable enough condition to support the weight of a jumbo jet.

I was on my own. The IDF had only allowed me one seat, so I couldn't bring a cameraman. In TV terminology, I was a one-man band. Instead, I packed a camera, batteries, laptop, charger, satellite transmitter, lights, stands, cables, clothes, and notepads into a few bags and boxes and hopped on the flight.

I found myself heading toward an inhospitable destination with no friends, about to face demons that I was not remotely ready to face. The moment I left Nepal, I knew I would one day return to thank my host family and the doctors who treated me. I also wanted to see with healthy eyes all that I had experienced as my body broke down. And I wanted to see our students again at the monastery.

But not like this. Not in the wake of a natural disaster, without Cassie, with my new job, and with our future on the line.

Let's backtrack a bit.

If you had asked me at any point during or immediately after our journey if I would be in this position, the answer would've been a resounding no. I don't mean about being on a humanitarian flight to Nepal following a devastating earthquake. I mean being a reporter in general.

When I left local TV news, I was absolutely convinced I was never getting back into news. I had had my fun being on TV, but I was ready for something new. Something different.

But something different was hard to find. Four months after we finished our trip, I was freelancing in public relations and video production, but I had yet to find a full-time job. We were living in Harlem, where Cassie was teaching English at a demanding but excellent charter school called Democracy Prep, which drew in students from Harlem, Queens, and the Bronx. We were definitely enjoying Big Apple life, but I was getting frustrated with the job hunt.

Out of nowhere, I landed an interview in December with CNN for an international correspondent position. They were looking for someone for Jerusalem or Beijing.

Frankly, I thought the interview was bullshit. Back in 2012, I had interviewed with CNN once for the Jerusalem position. My agent set up the interview when I told her I was thinking of quitting my job and traveling the world. No job means no money for her, so I suspect she called in a favor and set that interview up really quickly.

The interview was meaningless. It became evident ten minutes into the interview that they weren't serious about me. In return, I wasn't serious about them. Another interview with the same person felt like déjà vu.

Until it didn't. A few minutes in, as we talked about how much I enjoyed traveling the world and how much I loved both Jerusalem and Beijing, I realized they weren't kidding. They were serious. Very serious. This was for real. Beijing quickly dropped off the radar. We focused on Jerusalem.

As I shook hands with my interviewer, he said, "We'll try to get you back in here next week to meet more people. Let us know your schedule." The first interview hadn't ended anything like that.

He kept to his word. A week later, I was back in CNN's offices for another interview. A few weeks later, I was brought back to meet the top boss at CNN. And a day after that, I came in to meet the boss of CNN International.

I'll never forget that interview. It was January 12, 2015. The attacks at *Charlie Hebdo* and the kosher supermarket were the big story. In between following the latest updates, I was brushing up on the leadership of the Middle East. I felt fully prepared.

A second after walking in, the boss of CNN International hit me with a forceful spear of directness, blunted only slightly by his British accent.

"We've decided not to air the new *Charlie Hebdo* cover. What do you think about that?"

Great question. And I would've had a great answer had I ever actually seen the cover. Unfortunately for me, I hadn't. I was too busy all morning studying the latest developments in the Middle East to have a quick look at the planned *Charlie Hebdo* cover. (It showed a picture of Mohammed holding up a sign that reads, "I am Charlie.")

Even before the interview, I had heard stories about how quickly and ruthlessly this man sniffed out bovine excrement. He can spot bullshit even before you know you're planning it. In a very real and intimidating way, it is his superpower. And now it was directed at me. If I spat out even the slightest hint of bullshit, he would sense it and destroy me, or at least destroy my chances of landing a job at CNN.

Stuck in a corner with no other options, I committed fully to my only out. I spouted a line of bullshit.

"Well, you can argue it either way. There's no easy answer here, and you'll catch flak for whatever decision you make—airing the cover or not airing it." I kept going, all-in on an answer I was making up as I went.

Whatever answer I expressed confidently and without anything resembling a modicum of a clue, it worked. A few weeks later, I was in Atlanta for even more interviews. (Incidentally, when I saw him—then my new boss—a few months later, I told him about our exchange at the beginning of the interview. He didn't remember it but said it was a great question. I said, "Wonderful! I don't remember my answer, but I'm sure it was a great answer.")

A week later, CNN called to tell me they were going to offer me a job soon. This was great for two reasons: first, I would have a job, and second, we wouldn't have to cancel our trip to Panama the following week. Cassie and I had two trips on our agenda to keep our travel going: Panama in February and Scotland in April. I knew Scotland was out—we'd have to eat the price of the tickets—but it looked like we could still pull off the Panama trip, which suddenly took on new importance. It would be our last trip together before we spent a few months apart with the new job, and it would also mean that we would be overseas for the one-year anniversary of my diagnosis. It was a small but symbolic gesture that diabetes would never keep me from traveling.

I planned on making Cassie a nice dinner to celebrate—baked salmon with lemon dill sauce, sautéed spinach, and a good bottle of wine. As I started chopping the dill for the sauce, I looked away for a split second. Big mistake. With my razor sharp knife, I took off a chunk of the tip of my left index finger. One bandage didn't stop the bleeding. Neither did two. Or three. I pulled out gauze and wrapped my index finger. That helped, but only a little. Blood was everywhere. The bathroom looked like a crime scene. I had committed assault and battery against my finger. I eventually had to tourniquet my finger to stop the bleeding.

Cassie and I ordered takeout.

At least we were going to Panama!

While going through Panama immigration, I had to scan my fingers for security. Because of the partial finger-otomy I had performed on myself, my finger was wrapped in a few layers of cloth bandages. I could only scan nine fingers. By the time I left the country, my finger had healed and I could scan all ten. I really wonder what the immigration officials were thinking when they saw someone grow a new finger while in the country.

Why Panama?

First, why not? We found cheap tickets to a country we'd never visited. It was the only reason we need.

Second, we really wanted to see the Panama Canal. In Chile, we had visited Valparaiso, which was once the richest city in Latin America. Ships rounding the southern tip of South America had to stop in Valparaiso to resupply. The marine traffic made the city and its residents incredibly wealthy, driven by an economy focusing on trade. The Panama Canal destroyed this economy practically overnight. When it opened on August 15, 1914, there was suddenly no need to go all the way around South America, which meant no need to stop in Valparaiso. Having seen Valparaiso, we now wanted to see the canal to learn about the rest of the story.

Third, I love ceviche. And Panama has lots and lots of ceviche.

CNN offered me the job while we were in Boquete in northern Panama. I'll never forget the day because it was Ash Wednesday. Since Panama is a very Catholic country, everyone had ash in the shape of a cross on their foreheads. We had just been to a coffee plantation and on a birding hike, and the offer came in while we sat down for dinner. (We thought the birding hike was a waterfall tour—either way, it was quite fun and we got to see the quetzal, one of the rarest birds in the world.)

My new bosses asked via email if I could leave for London the following Thursday before heading to Jerusalem. Since I would get home on Sunday, that gave me four nights at home. I told them that would be fine.

Then another email came in. Could I be there Wednesday? Sure, no problem. What about Tuesday? Begrudgingly, yes. Then they sent me the tickets. I flew out Monday night. I would have one night at home.

To say that my one night at home was overwhelmingly hectic would be an understatement. I said goodbye to my parents and my in-laws, unpacked from Panama, packed for Jerusalem, sent off a bunch of emails, and tried to prepare myself for a new life overseas. Not a traveling life, but a "regular" life. Working during the week and having weekends off and that sort of thing.

I hopped on an overnight flight to begin my new job. After four days in London to meet my new bosses, I boarded a plane for Jerusalem. I had precisely one day off before I would be on-air. Prime Minister Benjamin Netanyahu's speech before the US Congress was on March 3, and I was providing the Israeli reaction. It kept me busy. That led into the elections, which transitioned into coalition building in the Israeli parliament, and that turned into the general chaos of reporting in the Middle East.

Then the earthquake hit. As soon as I heard rumors that Israel was sending a humanitarian mission, I tried to get on the flight, not really thinking about what it would mean for me personally or emotionally. I knew I wanted to make it to Pokhara if I could, but I also knew that wasn't likely, since I would be outrageously busy the moment I touched down.

I was absolutely right.

We land at two in the morning in Kathmandu. The airport looks like the kind of nightmare that makes civil aviation authorities snap awake at night drenched in cold sweat. People are everywhere, sprawled out among luggage that is equally spread out everywhere. It's impossible to tell who is coming and who is going, although it becomes quite clear that almost everyone at the airport will take the first flight to anywhere that is not here. It looks like more than a few people have been sleeping at the airport since the moments after the quake, hoping to catch any flight out that has a spare seat. Food wrappers and empty water bottles litter the floor. Everyone with a cell phone crowds around the few charging outlets available in the departures wing of the airport.

The Israeli flight that brought me in was on the ground less than two hours. It loaded up with a group of Israelis waiting to fly out and took off almost immediately. The soldiers and medical teams that flew in with me board buses and head straight for the site outside the city where they will set up a field hospital. I notice they carry with them a full-sized Torah in a protective case—not exactly a small piece of equipment. In a foreign country that is in desperate need of help, I suspect the Torah will bring them a spiritual peace in the midst of so much chaos. I'd bet many of the secular Israelis will pray as well. It will keep them grounded. Given the baggage I am carrying with me on this trip, I would need a new pancreas to keep me grounded.

Within thirty minutes of touching down, I am alone with my gear and a terminal full of foreigners, all of whom are trying to leave the country by any means possible. I do the only thing I can do. I start reporting.

I pull out my camera and roll on a few shots of the people at the airport. I set up all my gear and try to establish a satellite shot so I can go live. Since that's unsuccessful, I start doing live shots from my phone, using the breaks between lives to try to get in touch with our team on the ground in Kathmandu.

My demons are always lingering in the back of my mind. I remember how this airport feels and smells from the last time I was here—when I boarded a plane home after my diagnosis. I remember the departure wing. I remember the security check and the waiting area. And here I am again. Little things remind me of the time spent in Nepal. Little things that hit me in very powerful waves. An elderly woman hunched over, sweeping the floor with a bundle of straw, reminds me of Bimala cleaning the house. The taxi drivers cramming the arrivals hall reminds of my first entrance into this country.

At 10:00 a.m., a Nepali airport security guard approaches me outside the departures wing while I am trying, once again, to set up a live shot on the tarmac of the airport.

"Are you allowed to be here?"

"I've been here since two in the morning."

"Does anyone know you're here?"

"Yes, airport staff have seen me all morning here."

He walks off. After eight hours of me standing in the same spot with all of my equipment out, someone finally takes notice. Probably the new guy on the morning shift now that the overnight shift has gone home.

A few minutes later he returns with two more guards.

"You need to come with us now."

"What? Why?"

"You need to come with us now."

"Okay, give me a few minutes to put away my gear."

"You need to come with us now." I'm not sure he is trained to say anything else. I try to point out to him that I have a few thousand dollars of equipment that I am not going to leave there, but to no avail.

Admittedly, I am probably breaking a few rules. Broadcasting (or trying to broadcast) from the tarmac at an international airport without prior approval is generally frowned upon in every country on earth. But they've just had an earthquake, need all the help they could get, and I am attempting to show their problem to the world. I really think the guy has bigger problems to worry about.

Regardless, he drags me to the airport manager or head of security or something like that. Thankfully, this man is far more amenable to listening to reason.

"Hi. I'm with CNN. I just arrived a few hours ago with the Israeli humanitarian aid mission."

"Oh! You just arrived. Thank you for coming to report here. Welcome to Nepal."

He stamps my passport, gives me two minutes to pack all of my gear, and then promptly kicks me out of his airport.

It is perfect timing. My field producer and cameraman pick me up, and we keep working. We stay busy until midnight, shooting stories, grabbing interviews, and sending in photos. Late at night, I meet the field manager, make plans for the next day, and finally head to the hotel.

I hop in the shower to wash off a day of grime and sweat. I take a few deep breaths, and the baggage I've carried with me all day—the demons I have so far managed to avoid—hit me full force now that my defenses are down.

I had sworn that Laos would be the last time I'd shed any tears about diabetes. I break that vow. Heaving sobs rack my body as I gasp for air. Memories I'm not ready to face come flooding back. The moment of my diagnosis. My wait in the emergency room. The long nights in my hospital room. It all hits me, paralyzes me, incapacitates me.

Twenty minutes pass before I am finally able to regain some composure. An open window in the bathroom lets in some cold air—a welcome contrast to the scalding hot water of the shower.

I hop out of the shower, wrap myself in a towel, and lie down on the bed. Within moments, exhaustion overcomes me, and I am dead to the world. In a few hours, I will wake up and jump right into the relentless grind of news once again. In any rational way, I cannot connect the dots between us leaving to travel the world and me landing a job as CNN's Jerusalem correspondent. It doesn't make sense. A does not lead to B, and X definitely does not mark the spot. There is no sufficient explanation for how I've ended up with such an incredible job after throwing aside any chance of reasonable employment, waving goodbye to home, and being out of touch for a year. Somehow, it all just worked out for the best. And for that, I am eternally grateful.

Since my diagnosis, my blood sugar numbers have been great. Not perfect, but well within the healthy range. My HBA1C regularly falls between 5.6 and 5.8. I try to limit myself to dessert once every two weeks—easier said than done—and I generally try to eat healthy far more often than I used to. Diet Coke has become my vice of choice. I know it's not healthy, but there's a sweetness to it that keeps my desire for other sweets at bay.

Even after visiting some thirty countries, Cassie and I still long to travel. Since the official end of our trip, we have visited the Netherlands, Panama, Scotland, and Portugal. Sri Lanka and Cuba are now high on the list of places to visit next. When I was in Nepal, I didn't have a chance to see Krishna and Bimala or visit the doctors who treated me. For that reason, I know I will return to Nepal for a third time. I owe it to myself and to everyone I met there to see Nepal through healthy eyes, and I owe everyone a thank you. A thousand times over, thank you.

We miss life on the road. There's nothing like the freewheeling sense of adventure that comes from setting your own path every morning. But now we have someone else's path to set too.

On June 2, 2016, Cassie and I welcomed Noa Lillian into our lives. She weighed nine pounds and eleven ounces, and was easily the biggest baby in the nursery. She came out hungry as hell and ready to take on any other baby in the hospital. In short, she came out a Liebermann.

Because she was such a big baby, they had to regularly check her blood sugar to make sure she was getting enough food. The first time I saw this happen, I had to choke back tears. I knew she did not have diabetes, but it was still difficult to watch. In the back of my mind is the knowledge that she will have a higher probability of developing diabetes than other children. For that, I can blame no one but myself. I am the first person in my family with diabetes, and it would come from no one but me.

If that day ever comes, I know it will not be easy for me or Cassie or Noa. I will once again shed tears because of diabetes.

But I hope that if it does come, Noa will pick up this book and, somewhere within its pages, find inspiration.

Acknowledgments

If it takes a village to raise a child, it takes an army to write a book. There is much shouting of instructions, a fair amount of discipline, and sometimes you feel like you need just a few more tanks to complete the mission.

This book would not have been possible without the endless support of my wife, Cassie, both during our trip and every day since. (This book would also not be possible without my failed pancreas, but that mutinous organ is not getting any of my gratitude.)

Thank you to my wonderful agent, Joan, who guided me along this strange path since this book was no more than a collection of illegible notes in my trusty notepad. Thank you to Kim, Abigail, Jaidree, and the entire team at Skyhorse Publishing for taking a chance on this book. I cannot tell you how much I appreciate your help and support.

Of course, a huge thank you to the American Diabetes Association for their support and the work they do to advocate for the millions of us with diabetes and to educate the millions without. Your work will only get more important as the diabetes community grows.

I will always be indebted to my managers and colleagues at CNN who took a chance on me when I had been out of journalism for more than a year. A special thanks goes out to Sanjay, Elizabeth, Richard, Andrew, Michaela, and Mike for their help with this book.

Thank you to all of the reviewers who gave me input along the way. Patti, Jess, Richard, and so many others. Each of you made this book better with your critiques.

Thank you to my entire family for their love and support since long before I ever had the idea to write this book.

And naturally, thank you to anyone who picked up this book and gave it a shot. You had millions of other options for ways to pass your time, but for some reason, you ended up here. And I cannot express in any words I know how much I appreciate that.

See you on the road!

Appendix

American Diabetes Association

What is type 1 diabetes?

A diagnosis of type 1 diabetes means your pancreas is no longer capable of producing insulin. The body breaks down the sugars and starches you eat into a simple sugar called glucose, which it uses to fuel cells and give you the energy you need daily. Insulin is a hormone that the body needs to get glucose from the bloodstream into the cells of your body. Without insulin, glucose cannot enter your cells. Instead, it builds up in your blood system and can lead to potentially serious complications.

Type 1 diabetes is usually diagnosed in children and young adults, and it was previously known as juvenile diabetes. Approximately 1.25 million Americans have type 1 diabetes, roughly 5 percent of people with diabetes. Each year in the United States, an estimated 40,000 people are newly diagnosed.

People living with diabetes manage their blood glucose levels through an important balance of food, exercise, and medication. If you have type 1 diabetes, insulin is required. The goal of treatment is to come as close to mimicking the normal action of the pancreas of a person that does not have diabetes. Although this is challenging for the person and, at times, the loved ones whose support is important, a growing number of people are living the fullest of lives with type 1 diabetes. To balance diabetes at more optimal levels, it is necessary to monitor blood glucose levels using a blood glucose monitor several or more times a day and night, or use a continuous glucose monitor (CGM) and administer the right amount of insulin to keep your glucose levels in your target range. You need to work closely with your diabetes healthcare team to determine which insulin or insulins are best for you and your body. With a tailored insulin therapy program, a solid understanding and consumption of healthy foods, and enough exercise and other treatments if needed, even young children do learn to manage their condition and enjoy long, healthy lives.

The ADA's diabetes camps and retreats offer unique opportunities for children and their families to gain unique peer support and friendships while working with knowledgeable diabetes professionals and recreation staff who often have diabetes themselves and who serve as influential positive role models that last a lifetime.

Type 1 Diabetes Symptoms
The following symptoms of diabetes are typical. Common symptoms include:
- Urinating often
- Feeling very thirsty
- Feeling very hungry—even though you are eating
- Extreme fatigue
- Blurry vision
- Cuts/bruises that are slow to heal
- Weight loss—even though you are may be eating and drinking more

I've been diagnosed with type 1 diabetes.
Now, what do I do?
You've just been told you have type 1 diabetes, now what? Understanding diabetes and its effects, both near term and long term, is very important. Education and emotional support is key for you and your loved ones. Talk with your primary care physician regarding your next steps. She will refer you to an endocrinologist, a specialist in blood and hormone disorders and treatment. He will help you find a good health care team, typically nurses and dietitians who are trained diabetes educators and who will help you understand what you must do on a daily basis to control your type 1 diabetes and maintain a healthy lifestyle.

We encourage you to seek additional information online at www.diabetes.org/type1 or contact or call us at 1-800-DIABETES (800-342-2383), Monday through Friday, 8:30 a.m. to 8:00 p.m. Eastern Time.

Who is on my health care team?

Your health care team should consist of everyone you need to help you understand your type 1 diabetes and what to do on a daily basis. It typically includes your physician who is either an endocrinologist or a primary care physician who has a special understanding of type 1 diabetes. Your diabetes specialist will prescribe the type and amount of insulin(s), any technologies if needed/desired (insulin pens, insulin pumps, and continuous glucose monitors [CGM]), and other medications you might need based on blood sugar, as well as any other needed lab results. Optimally, your diabetes specialty team should include along with your physician: a registered nurse or nurse practitioner, a registered dietitian, a psychologist, and access to someone who understands diabetes and exercise. This team will help you understand your insulin(s); glucose monitoring techniques and how to interpret blood sugar results; how to balance your insulin(s) with food, exercise, and schedules; and how to share relevant information about your diabetes with others and build your support network of family, friends, and peers. Your diabetes team members are available to help you and your loved ones navigate diagnosis and guide you towards your new normal.

What can I eat now?

There is no such thing as a "diabetes diet." Healthy, balanced nutrition is a very important part of managing your type 1 diabetes. Knowing how the foods you eat affect you and your diabetes balance will help you plan your meals and insulin delivery for the day. Living with diabetes requires more planning, and with proper planning you can enjoy life to the fullest.

Counting Carbs

The keys to balanced nutrition are understanding carbohydrates and knowing the right portions for you. All foods are made up of carbohydrate, protein, and fat. Carbohydrates have the greatest effect on your blood glucose levels. And, carbohydrates are in most of the foods you eat. So, it is important that you can recognize foods high in carbohydrates and are able to estimate their amount. It's also helpful to know the best sources of lean pro-tein. All protein contains some fat, but some protein foods, such as salmon, tuna, sardines, and herring, contain beneficial fats. Learning about adjust-ing insulin for high-fat meals is an individualized but important concept. There are many websites and books that can help you understand meal planning and carbohydrate counting, such as:

"What Can I Eat," ADA (http://www.diabetes.org/what-can-i-eat/) *What Do I Eat Now?*, 2nd edition (*ADA Books, ISBN* 978-1-58040-558-4)

Know Your Portions
It is no secret that all too often portion sizes in the United States are too large for most people. One way to get your bearings and use a visual aid is—the portion plate. Using a standard dinner plate with a nine-inch diam-eter, divide the plate as follows:

- Make a quarter of your plate a protein-rich food (for example: a lean meat, chicken, or fish; beans; eggs or cheese)
- Make another quarter of your plate grains or starchy food (for example: green peas, sweet potato, brown rice, quinoa)
- Make half of your plate non-starchy vegetables (for example: carrots, broccoli, spinach, or peppers)

See http://www.diabetes.org/create-your-plate for more information on better portions.

Lifestyle Changes

Physical Activity
Regular activity is a key part of managing diabetes along with meal plan-ning, taking medications as prescribed, and stress management. When you are active, your cells become more sensitive to insulin so it can work more efficiently. So, exercising consistently can help lower blood glucose levels, reduce weight (if this is a goal), and improve your A1C, an average measure of blood glucose levels. When you lower your A1C, you will keep your body healthier today and for your many tomorrows. Physical activity is also important for your overall wellbeing and can help with many other health conditions.

Benefits of regular physical activity:
- lowers blood pressure and cholesterol
- lowers your risk for heart disease and stroke
- helps you lose or maintain weight
- increases your energy for daily activities
- helps you sleep better
- relieves stress
- strengthens your heart and improves your blood circulation
- strengthens your muscles and bones
- keeps your joints flexible
- improves your balance to prevent falls
- reduces symptoms of depression
- improves quality of life

You can experience these benefits even if you haven't been very active before.

Types of Activity
Aerobic exercise, strength training, flexibility exercises/stretching, balance exercises, and activity throughout the day are the types of activities we recommend for people with diabetes.

Visit http://www.diabetes.org/physical-activity for more information and activities.

Travel
Learning to manage your type 1 diabetes when traveling can seem daunting, but it is easier than you think. Whether you are traveling by automobile, train, ship, or plane—for business or pleasure—it requires planning and organization.

Tips for packing
- Take enough supplies and medication for your trip, plus extras in case you are delayed.
- Make sure all your diabetes supplies are in a bag you carry with you.
- Pack extra snacks (and glucose tablets) in your carry-on bag.

- If traveling by plane, put your insulin in your carry-on bag. The luggage compartments of airplanes can be very cold and your insulin could freeze. Or, your luggage may be left out in the hot sun.
- If you use an insulin pump, take an alternative source of insulin and insulin delivery (syringes or insulin pens with needles) in case your pump stops working while you are away. The larger pump companies have an emergency number on the back of their pumps that you can call if your pump is not working properly.
- When traveling overseas, ask your diabetes team if they have a diabetes contact in the country you are going to visit.

Carry-on bag checklist
Medications
- Insulin or other injectable medications or pens
- Syringes, pen needles, pump supplies, CGM supplies
- Oral diabetes medications
- Glucose tablets or another source of quick-acting carbohydrate
- Snacks, such as dried fruit or crackers
- Antibiotic ointment
- Other prescribed medications
- Glucagon kit
- Anti-nausea and anti-diarrhea medications

Blood Monitoring Equipment
- Enough test strips for your trip and unexpected delays
- Lancets
- Blood sampling device and a spare
- Glucose meter
- Hand-washing gel or alcohol wipes
- Spare batteries for glucose meter, continuous glucose monitor (CGM)
- Cotton or tissues

General Tips
- Wear a medical ID bracelet or necklace that says you have diabetes.

- Keep a prescription for insulin and other medications on hand, just in case.
- Always pack more diabetes medications and supplies in case of emergencies and delays.
- Don't get separated from your supplies.

Security Checkpoints

Your diabetes equipment and medications are necessary and permitted through security checkpoints; however, it is wise to check for new rules and requirements issued by security agencies (for example, the US Transportation Security Administration [TSA]) to ensure there are no surprises during your trip. Carry a written prescription signed by your physician that says you may purchase and carry each of your diabetes medications and supplies.

Visit: http://www.diabetes.org/traveltips.

Meals While Traveling

Planning meals is an important part of your trip. If traveling by plane or train, many flights or travel segments do not offer food service. It is critical to bring or purchase a nutritious meal or meals with you to eat on your needed schedule. If you have arranged for a special meal in flight or while riding the train, remember that you may not want to inject your pre-meal insulin until your meal has been served as sometimes there are significant delays.

Traveling Across Time Zones

Adjusting insulin injections for time zones can be a major challenge. When traveling from west to east, you lose hours from your day, and you may need less insulin. When traveling from east to west, you will add hours to your day, and you may need extra insulin. If you are uncertain of how to plan your insulin and meals, take a copy of your itinerary and work schedule to your diabetes health care team and get their advice.

Who is the American Diabetes Association?

For more than seventy-five years, the American Diabetes Association has created and provided state-of-the-art information about all aspects of diabetes. The moving force behind the work of the Association is a network of more than one million volunteers; a membership of more than 500,000 people with diabetes, their families, and caregivers; and a professional society of nearly 14,000 health care professionals; as well as more than 800 staff members.

We lead the fight against the deadly consequences of diabetes and fight for those affected by diabetes.

- We fund research to prevent, cure, and manage diabetes.
- We deliver services to hundreds of communities.
- We provide objective and credible information.
- We give voice to those denied their rights because of diabetes. Learn more at: http://www.diabetes.org/.

American Diabetes Association
2451 Crystal Drive, Suite 900
Arlington, VA 22202
1-800-DIABETES (800-342-2383)
http://diabetes.org
http://www.diabetes.org/type1/

Again, don't forget to discuss your diabetes needs with your diabetes team. Often, they will be your best advisors.

(February 15, 2017)